What we sh... ...ut

GW01418194

HIV & AIDS

What we should all know about HIV & AIDS
Second edition

Written and edited by:
Dr Martin Fisher
The Elton John Centre, Brighton General Hospital, Brighton

in conjunction with:
Dr Graham P Taylor
Imperial College School of Medicine, St Mary's Hospital, London

Stephen Head, Clinical Nurse Specialist and Jo White, Specialist
Health Visitor, Family Clinic, St. Mary's Hospital, London

Fatima Patel and Heather Simmonds, Mediscript Ltd

Endorsed by the British HIV Association (BHIVA)

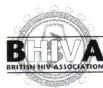

What we should all know about HIV & AIDS
is published by

Mediscript
1 Mountview Court
310 Friern Barnet Lane
London N20 0LD
UK

This publication has been supported by educational grants from:
DuPont Pharma
Merck Sharp & Dohme

Contents

The **acquired immune deficiency syndrome** (AIDS) was first recognised in 1981 when groups of homosexual men in the United States were noted to develop unusual infections and cancers. AIDS is the term used when an individual has developed one (or more) of a number of specific infections or tumours that are the result of damage to the immune system.

The causative virus, the **human immunodeficiency virus** (HIV), was discovered in 1983. If you are infected with the virus, you are HIV-positive. Nevertheless, you may feel completely well and not have any related illnesses. Thus, HIV infection and the illness AIDS are not the same, although they are considered to be two extremes of the same illness.

Origins

HIV seems to have been present in the human population for many years before it was recognised. Cases of HIV infection have been traced back at least to the 1950s. Although there is a continuing scientific debate about the exact origins of the virus, many scientists believe that HIV evolved from a similar animal virus in monkeys in Central Africa.

Increasing significance for individuals and countries

Globally, the number of cases of HIV infection and AIDS continues to rise at an alarming rate. Since many cases are unrecognised, it is difficult to give precise figures for those affected, but it is clear that many millions of people around the world are infected.

Recent developments in the management of HIV infection have dramatically altered the outlook for many individuals with HIV, although a number of important issues remain unclear. While newer treatments have significantly extended the life of many patients, especially in the developed world, they have also brought new problems, including side effects of the drugs and development of drug-resistant strains of HIV. As yet, there is no evidence that HIV can be eliminated from the body once the infection has been acquired.

This book aims to explain what HIV and AIDS are, how HIV infection is currently treated, how individuals may protect themselves from infection and to provide some general information on living with HIV. A comprehensive coverage of these issues is beyond the scope of this book, and since scientific knowledge in this field has been growing very rapidly indeed in recent years, some of the information provided will quickly be superseded. Nonetheless, the basic outline provided here will lead to a better understanding of HIV and its treatment, allowing more informed discussions with healthcare providers and HIV/AIDS agencies.

2 The virus and the immune system

HIV is one of a family of viruses called retroviruses that contain their genetic material or chromosomes in a form called RNA. In contrast, humans, animals, bacteria and most other viruses have DNA chromosomes.

Structurally, HIV is a simple virus composed of a sugar-protein surface and a protein core surrounding an eight-gene RNA chromosome. Structures on the surface of the virus enable it to bind to certain human cells. Specifically, the virus attaches to and infects cells of the human immune system; the most notable of these are the CD4 (T-helper or T4) lymphocytes, which are important in coordinating the body's response against infection.

The structure of HIV is shown in Figure 1.

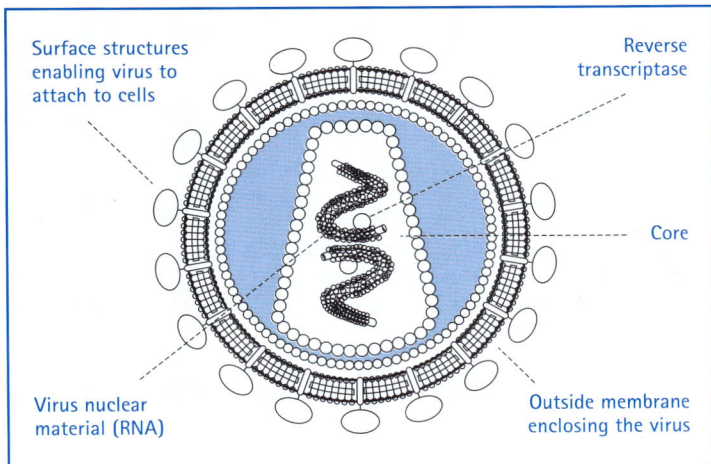

Figure 1: Structure of HIV.

Mode of attack

When the virus enters a cell, it converts its RNA chromosome into DNA using its unique enzyme reverse transcriptase. Once formed into double-stranded DNA, the virus can become integrated into a human chromosome, where it remains for the life of the cell. This cell is called the host cell as it is 'playing host' to the integrated virus.

Using the genetic machinery of the host cell, the viral chromosome can be copied and new immature viruses produced. These immature forms of the virus are released through the membrane of the human cell, after which they mature rapidly using a viral enzyme called protease. The virus is now ready to infect another human cell.

This life cycle is shown in Figure 2.

The integrated viral material is initially 'active', causing the cell to produce multiple new HIV particles. Subsequently, the integrated viral material may lie 'dormant' (without producing new viruses) indefinitely or may have bursts of activity that are brought on by certain activities within its host cell, for example in response to certain other infections. If the virus becomes very active in its host cell, it may cause the host cell to split open, thus killing the cell.

The immune system

The human immune system protects the body against infections and tumours. It is made up of many different cells in different parts of the body, each of which serves different purposes and many of which can move around the body as necessary. These cells can communicate with one another by chemical messengers or can respond to the presence of 'foreign' objects such as bacteria or other infectious organisms. Some cells produce antibodies, which attach to infectious particles, while others bind to such particles and attack them.

The CD4 cells (sometimes called T-4 or T-helper cells) help to co-ordinate the way in which these different cells communicate with one another, and hence the way in which the body responds to infection.

How the immune system responds to HIV

After infection with HIV, the human body mounts a strong immune response against the virus by activating specific cells:

◆ Suppressor cells (called CD8 lymphocytes) kill HIV-infected cells and can produce chemicals that reduce new HIV production.

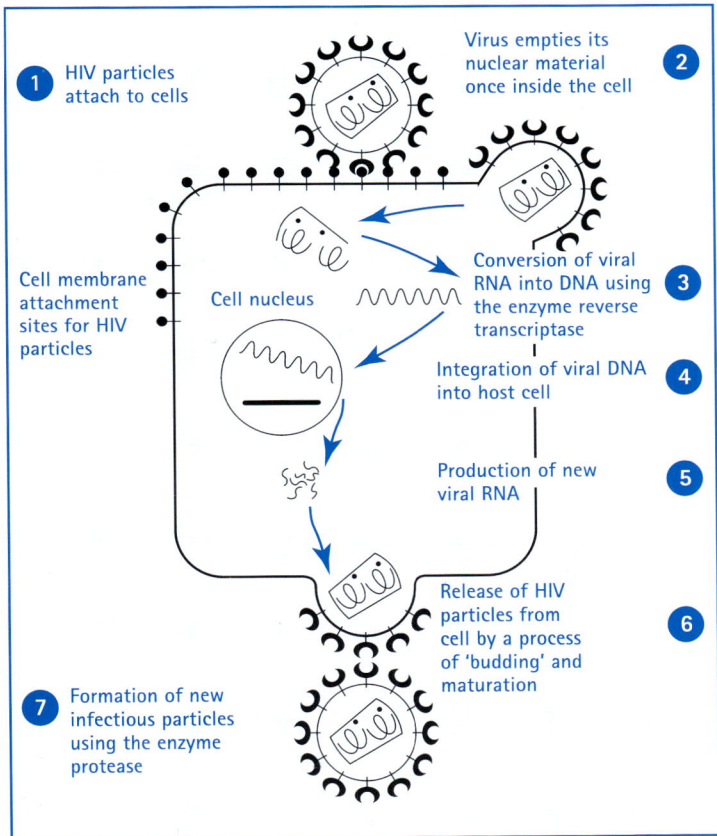

Figure 2: Life cycle of HIV, shown in stages.

◆ Antibodies are produced by B lymphocytes, which can bind to HIV particles and reduce their ability to infect new cells.

These immune responses may limit the infection for a period of time, but the virus is able to escape from the cells and antibodies and, as the immune system becomes damaged, these responses become weaker and are insufficient to prevent new HIV particles being formed or new cells becoming infected.

How HIV damages the immune system

HIV infects the CD4 cells (as shown in Figure 2). These can then be destroyed by several mechanisms:

◆ High levels of HIV turnover can cause the cells to burst.
◆ Groups of infected and uninfected CD4 cells can clump together, and all then die.
◆ CD8 cells may kill infected CD4 cells or produce chemicals that kill them.

Since the CD4 cells have a co-ordinating role in the immune system, the entire system functions less and less well as these cells are increasingly damaged and destroyed.

Epidemiology

Epidemiology is the study of disease in relation to populations; it provides information on how the spread of a disease has developed, where it is now and how it is likely to spread in the future.

Since the first reported cases of AIDS in 1981, the number of cases of HIV infection and AIDS in the world have grown from a relatively isolated phenomenon affecting a small subset of the population to a global disease affecting all social classes.

The AIDS epidemic has evolved into a pandemic. This means that the disease, which has already affected a large number of people in particular areas (epidemic), has now become widespread over an exceptionally large area, that is, across continents (pandemic).

The global figures for HIV infection continue to grow at an alarming rate. These figures are likely to underestimate the true picture quite considerably, since many people are not aware of their HIV status and reporting mechanisms around the world vary in accuracy. However, estimates from the World Health Organization (WHO) suggest that 34.3 million men, women and children worldwide were living with HIV/AIDS in June 2000 (Figure 3). An estimated 5.4 million new infections occurred during 1999 alone (Figure 4). A record number of people died of AIDS and AIDS-related diseases in 1999: an estimated 2.6 million people, mostly in the developing nations.

In the United Kingdom, cumulative figures to March 1999 showed 37,875 cases of HIV infection, 16,201 cases of AIDS and 13,017 deaths. However, as in other Western countries, the rate of new infections appears to be falling, and the annual number of new AIDS cases peaked in 1994, falling most dramatically in 1998, with the introduction of new treatments. Nevertheless, HIV remains a challenge in industrialised countries, with new infections occurring consistently, many individuals being unaware of their HIV status and because new treatments may not be effective or manageable

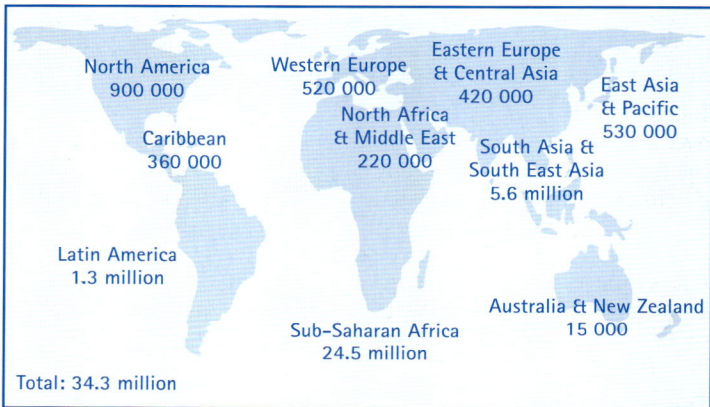

Figure 3: Number of adults and children estimated to be living with HIV and AIDS, June 2000 (Source: World Health Organization, Geneva).

North America
900 000

Western Europe
520 000

Eastern Europe
& Central Asia
420 000

East Asia
& Pacific
530 000

North Africa
& Middle East
220 000

Caribbean
360 000

South Asia &
South East Asia
5.6 million

Latin America
1.3 million

Australia & New Zealand
15 000

Sub-Saharan Africa
24.5 million

Total: 34.3 million

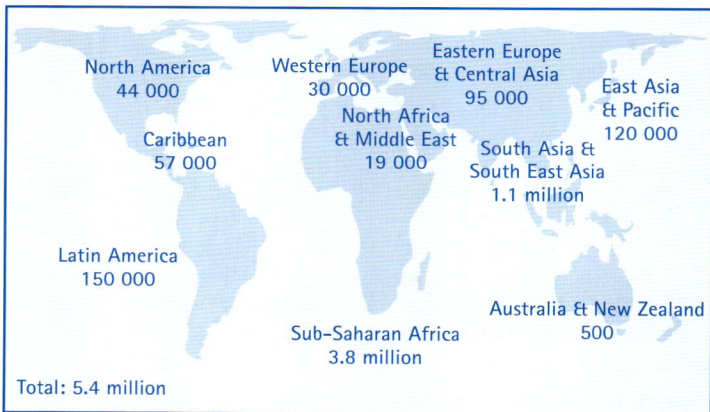

Figure 4: Estimated number of new HIV infections occurring in adults and children during 1999 (Source: World Health Organization, Geneva).

North America
44 000

Western Europe
30 000

Eastern Europe
& Central Asia
95 000

East Asia
& Pacific
120 000

North Africa
& Middle East
19 000

Caribbean
57 000

South Asia &
South East Asia
1.1 million

Latin America
150 000

Australia & New Zealand
500

Sub-Saharan Africa
3.8 million

Total: 5.4 million

for all patients. In addition, there is some concern that safe sexual behaviour may be relaxed by the perception that life-prolonging therapy is now available.

In the early 1980s, HIV and AIDS were predominantly recognised in homosexual men, haemophiliacs and intravenous drug users.

However, in subsequent years, it became apparent that HIV is not restricted to any individual risk groups and can affect anyone irrespective of sexuality, sex, race or drug-using practices.

The pattern of groups affected varies from country to country and over time. In the UK, where infections were initially diagnosed in the communities identified above, the number of reported cases in heterosexuals is increasing with time (although in many cases such individuals have either lived in or travelled to areas with high rates of infection). In sub-Saharan Africa and the Indian subcontinent, the HIV epidemic has predominantly affected the heterosexual population. Globally, heterosexuals account for the majority of cases of HIV and AIDS, with men and women infected in equal numbers.

Transmission

It is very easy to become infected with some viruses, such as chickenpox and the common cold: these viruses can be transmitted by air to someone near an infected individual who inhales viral particles from the patient's exhaled air. However, HIV cannot be transmitted by everyday social contact.

The body fluids of an infected person that can transmit HIV infection are:

◆ blood;
◆ semen;
◆ vaginal and cervical secretions; and
◆ breast milk.

There are three ways in which HIV can be transmitted from one person to another. These are:

◆ sexual intercourse (vaginal, anal and, possibly, oral);
◆ exposure to blood (by injection or transfusion); and
◆ from mother to baby (in the womb or via breast milk).

HIV cannot be transmitted by:

◆ caring for people with HIV;
◆ social contact among people with HIV;
◆ sharing cutlery, plates or cups;
◆ using the same toilet as someone with HIV;
◆ swimming pools, showers or washing machines;

- ◆ mouth-to-mouth resuscitation;
- ◆ animal bites; or
- ◆ mosquito bites.

Rarely, the virus has been transmitted through the mouth (if there are cuts, sores or bleeding gums) or the eyes (if splashed with large amounts of blood). It is best not to share toothbrushes and razors.

Sexual intercourse

HIV infection can occur when men have unprotected sexual intercourse with women or other men. Women who have sexual intercourse with other women appear to have less risk from infection or transmission.

Sexual transmission of HIV occurs through both vaginal and anal sexual intercourse. Cases of transmission through oral intercourse have also been reported. The likely risk of transmission by oral sex is very much smaller than for anal or vaginal sex, but may be increased if there is ejaculation, bleeding gums or sores, or inflammation caused by common throat infections or sexually transmitted diseases. Some sexual activities appear to be more dangerous than others; for example, anal intercourse is thought to transmit HIV more easily than any other activity. In addition, sores or ulcers on the genital area break the body's defences and allow viruses to invade more easily. The presence of a sexually transmitted infection in either partner is likely to increase the risk of transmission.

On a worldwide basis, unprotected sexual intercourse is the main means by which HIV is transmitted from person to person.

Exposure to blood

Injecting virus through the skin is another method of transmission. This type of transmission is a particular risk to those who inject drugs and share needles with other injecting drug users.

Blood transfusions or infusions of special proteins made from donated blood (such as the use of Factor VIII to treat haemophilia) provided another concern before sensitive antibody tests for HIV became available. In industrialised countries, all blood and blood products are now screened carefully for HIV (since 1985) and are not used if there is the slightest concern about their being an infection risk. Blood products in other, less developed countries may not be so safe.

From mother to baby

Transmission of HIV from a positive mother to her baby can occur in three ways:

◆ in the uterus (womb);
◆ at birth; and
◆ by breast-feeding.

It seems that babies born of HIV-infected mothers are often infected at the time of birth rather than during pregnancy. Treatment with anti-HIV drugs, delivery by Caesarian section, and avoidance of breast-feeding may all help to reduce the chances of transmission (see Chapter 10).

Avoiding infection

HIV-infected people may appear completely healthy, may not be aware of their infection and may, therefore, unwittingly transmit HIV to others. If you are not infected, you should take measures to protect yourself, and if you are infected, you should be careful not to infect others. There is a theoretical risk of re-infection with HIV (which may be drug-resistant), and even if both partners are HIV-positive, the same concerns may apply.

Sexual activity

'Safer sex' is the term given to activities associated with a low risk of transmitting HIV. Such activities include:

◆ oral sex (without ejaculation);
◆ using sex toys.

Many people will wish to have penetrative intercourse. The risk of transmission of HIV during intercourse may be reduced by both physical and chemical barriers, and may be increased by injuries or infections that damage the protective barriers provided by our body surfaces.

Condoms are simple to use, widely available and excellent barriers to the transmission of both HIV and other sexually transmitted diseases. However, they do not provide 100% protection, because they can occasionally break or slip off during use, frequently due to incorrect usage. The following tips should reduce this:

◆ Practise before using.
◆ Choose a strong brand.

◆ Use a water-based lubricant (not oil-based).

◆ Store condoms properly (not in hot places).

◆ Do not re-use.

Spermicides are chemicals that kill sperm and are used alone, as contraceptives, or to improve the effectiveness of barrier contraceptives, such as diaphragms and condoms. In a laboratory setting, spermicides kill all viruses, including HIV. However, it has not been proved that spermicides reduce the chances of acquiring HIV. Indeed, nonoxynol-9 appears to be an irritant to some women, a factor that may increase the chances of HIV transmission. Therefore, spermicidal agents and carriers, including the 'sponge', should NOT be regarded as protection against HIV.

The recently introduced female condom (femidom) is based on similar principles to those of the male condom and may provide women with a greater opportunity to take control of establishing safer sex. Some people have also used the femidom for anal sex.

The most sensible approach to safer sex and personal protection against HIV is to use a condom every time, with every partner. This involves being prepared by always carrying condoms and being determined either to practise safer sex or not to have penetrative sexual intercourse. This can be awkward and embarrassing, and you may think that a relationship that you care about could be put at risk; however, practising safer sex with your new partner shows how much you care about both yourself and your partner, and removes anxieties about HIV and other sexually transmitted diseases. Some couples in regular relationships may choose to have HIV tests together and to stop using condoms if both test negative. If you decide to adopt this strategy, you must understand the limitations of HIV testing (see Chapter 4) and you need to be clear about other relationships.

Risk from blood, blood products and other medical procedures

As blood and blood products are tested for HIV in most industrialised countries, receiving a transfusion is no longer considered to present a risk of HIV infection.

Donated blood in the United Kingdom is very safe because of the HIV tests that are used and because blood donors are asked not to donate if they are at high risk of being infected with HIV. However, in some less affluent nations, there may not be the facilities for adequate testing for HIV infection and donated blood remains a possible source of infection. When travelling abroad, avoid blood transfusion unless it is a matter of life or death. Any traveller should try to ensure that blood is tested for HIV before receiving a transfusion and that sterile equipment is used to administer any treatment. Some travel clinics sell specialised travel health kits to help reduce the risk of HIV infection from poorly sterilised medical equipment. Such kits include a selection of needles, syringes, cannulae for drips and surgical thread. This can reduce the risk of exposure to potentially infected needles if medical treatment is required abroad.

Intravenous drug users

Sharing infected needles can lead to the spread of HIV as well as to the spread of hepatitis viruses, such as hepatitis B and hepatitis C. For those injecting recreational drugs, safe practices have been developed. These involve:

◆ not sharing injecting equipment (either needles or syringes);

◆ disposing of needles in puncture-proof containers; and

◆ using clean injecting equipment every time.

The availability of needle-exchange centres has made the use of clean equipment possible in many cities; where none is available, rinsing injecting equipment with bleach after use will destroy any HIV present.

Extremely low risk from infected healthcare workers

The consensus is that the average doctor or nurse is more at risk of HIV infection from their patients than vice versa. Although there has been considerable concern about the possibility of HIV-infected healthcare workers infecting their patients, all statistics suggest that this risk is extremely low.

An HIV-infected dentist in Florida, USA, was blamed for infecting some of his patients. This outbreak was investigated extensively, but is still not fully understood. Dentists, like all healthcare workers, are now required to maintain strict infection control procedures, which should prevent any similar episode occurring.

A doctor or a nurse infected with HIV is only a risk to a patient if the patient is undergoing an invasive medical procedure and is contaminated accidentally with the doctor's or nurse's blood. Healthcare workers wear gloves for all such procedures, and so the only risk appears to be from a doctor who receives a cut from a sharp instrument during surgery.

There is only one established case of a doctor transmitting HIV to a patient. A surgeon in France transmitted HIV during a lengthy operation in 1983 while unaware of his own HIV status. Despite numerous 'look-back' exercises involving thousands of patients, no other case has been discovered anywhere in the world. Doctors in the United Kingdom who perform major surgical procedures are required to seek advice if they are worried that they may have HIV infection and, if found to be HIV-positive, are re-trained in a less invasive branch of medicine.

Post-exposure prophylaxis

It is believed, although there is little clear evidence, that healthcare workers exposed to HIV from patients (by needlestick injuries or significant blood splashes) are less likely to become infected if they take anti-HIV therapy after the accident. Therefore, a 4-week course of anti-HIV drugs is recommended to healthcare workers who incur high-risk injuries. However, this therapy is complex, has many side effects and needs to be started as soon as possible after the injury.

To date, there is no evidence to say whether this approach may be helpful after high-risk sexual activity. Many clinics have given therapy in this situation but few would recommend it routinely. If you and your partner have different HIV test results, it may be worth discussing what you should do if an accident (e.g. a condom breakage) occurs, before it happens. Your doctor should be happy to discuss this situation with you and outline the risks and benefits of post-exposure therapy. However, because many unpleasant side effects may occur, you cannot use this treatment as a 'morning after pill' to avoid the need for safer sexual practices.

What is an HIV test?

An HIV test is a blood test that looks for antibodies in the bloodstream which indicate whether an individual has been infected with HIV. It is not an AIDS test; the diagnosis of AIDS is based on the presence of particular illnesses (see Chapter 5).

Antibodies to HIV are produced 4–12 weeks after infection. These antibodies can be detected in a variety of body fluids, including blood, saliva, spinal fluid and vaginal secretions. As detection of antibodies to HIV in the blood is the most sensitive method of easily identifying the presence of HIV, the HIV test is normally performed on blood. It tests for antibodies produced by the body in response to infection by HIV and is a very sensitive and specific method of detecting infection by the virus. Antibodies cannot be produced by the body unless infection has occurred.

Since antibody production occurs after infection, there is a short period when you may test negative even when you are infected with HIV. This can happen if the HIV test is performed within about 3 months of infection, which is often termed the 'window period'.

If you are worried about an activity that happened more than 3 months before having an HIV test, the test will tell you whether you have been infected or not. If you are worried about an episode within the last 3 months, the test may not be helpful and you may choose to test at a later time point or discuss the matter with an appropriate healthcare worker.

How and where?

HIV tests are free of charge (in the United Kingdom) and can be performed at a hospital clinic (sexually transmitted disease or genito-urinary medicine clinic) or by your general practitioner. Many hospital clinics have open access and no appointment is necessary; however, you will require an appointment at some clinics and it is best to telephone in advance. Many clinics offer results on the same day as your blood is taken; an appointment is usually required for this service.

Many people prefer to have HIV tests performed anonymously at a hospital clinic, where no information about you is passed to your general practitioner (GP) without your consent. Others prefer to have a test with a family doctor whom they know well. This decision is yours.

What will happen?

If you attend a hospital clinic, you will usually be seen by a doctor, nurse or health adviser, who will discuss the issues with you, including the nature of the test, your possible risks of exposure, the advantages and disadvantages of testing, who you should or shouldn't tell and when to return for the result. You may well be recommended to undergo tests for other sexually transmitted infections as well. You may wish to do this at the same time or to return after your HIV result.

Should you have one?

For everyone, there will be different issues around HIV testing. You should discuss these fully before deciding whether or not testing is right for you or whether this is the right time to test. The staff at clinics will be more than happy to discuss these questions with you.

Reasons for having a test

Some reasons why you might have an HIV test are that:

◆ knowing that you are HIV-positive may encourage you to practice safer sex, and thus reduce the risk of your partner becoming infected or encourage you to stop sharing needles if you inject drugs;

◆ finding that you are HIV-negative may be a relief if you have been very worried but did not know your status before;

◆ knowing that you are HIV-positive enables you to have treatment that may give you a longer life than if you were not treated and reduce illnesses;

◆ knowing that you are HIV-positive assists in the diagnosis and management of HIV-associated infections;

◆ women who are pregnant or considering becoming pregnant may plan their pregnancy to ensure that the chances of the child becoming HIV-positive can be minimised;

- knowing that you are HIV-positive allows you to adopt non-medical changes to prevent your health from deteriorating;
- knowing that you are HIV-positive may allow you to plan ahead and do things that you may not otherwise have done;
- many people find that knowing their status (even if positive) is not as bad as the uncertainty of not knowing whether one is positive or negative.

Reasons for not having a test

Some of the reasons why you might not want to have an HIV test are:

- concerns about employment if HIV-positive;
- fears of stigmatisation if HIV-positive;
- concerns over housing and mortgage issues;
- worries about sexual and social isolation; and
- concerns over confidentiality.

You may find that many of these fears are reduced after you have discussed them at the clinic/surgery before deciding to test. It is now widely believed that with the new developments in HIV therapy, on balance, a person who is HIV-positive is likely have a better quality of life and/or a longer life if treated for the infection.

What will happen when I get the result?

You will usually have arranged a time to return for your result. You will be given one of three answers: negative, positive or indeterminate.

A negative test

A negative test result will mean that no antibodies to HIV have been found. This will not necessarily mean that you do not have HIV if you have been at risk within the past 3 months (as outlined above). If your result is negative, you may want to seek advice from one of the clinic team on how to negotiate safer sex. They will also discuss with you methods for reducing the chances of your becoming infected with other sexually transmitted diseases (such as hepatitis A and B). You should be aware that if you test negative, this does not automatically imply that your sexual partner is also negative.

A positive test

A positive test result will mean that antibodies to HIV have been found, showing that you have been infected with HIV. At that point, you will be offered further support, including referral to an appropriate specialist for medical care and advice on any problems arising from the diagnosis. Healthcare professionals will be available to discuss methods by which you may be helped to inform those close to you and to arrange further counselling if you wish. The blood test will also be repeated to confirm the result. It is not usually possible to tell from blood tests when, how or from whom the infection was acquired.

An indeterminate test

Rarely, the result may return as 'equivocal' or 'indeterminate'; this means that it is not entirely clear whether you have been infected or not. In this situation, a further blood test will be performed and more complex testing done to clarify the situation. In this unusual situation, your healthcare worker will guide you through what is being done.

5 Spectrum of the disease

What to expect with HIV infection and AIDS

The period of time from acquisition of HIV to the onset of associated illnesses is very variable. Without treatment of any sort, at least 50% of people infected with HIV will develop one of the diseases that constitute AIDS within 10 years. For much of this time, the infected individual may feel completely healthy and may be unaware of the infection and of the danger of infecting others. Many, however, experience symptoms that reflect a decline in the immune system and, although the time frame for this decline is variable, it is described frequently in the stages summarised below.

Seroconversion illness

A glandular fever-like illness may develop 4–6 weeks after infection. This is termed 'seroconversion illness' because it corresponds with the time that the serum or blood converts from being negative to being positive for HIV antibodies. Seroconversion illness, which is usually mild, is characterised by enlarged lymph nodes, sore throat and fever. Those who experience a more severe case of seroconversion illness may complain of a rash and diarrhoea. A minority of people at this stage develop impaired immune systems, but most recover completely from this acute illness and appear to be healthy for many years.

While this may be the optimal time for anti-HIV therapy to preserve the immune system in as normal a state as possible, it may be very difficult to start a complex treatment regimen almost immediately after learning you are HIV-positive. Most clinicians suggest that anyone who has symptoms of seroconversion and/or has experienced a significant risk in the previous 3 months should rapidly consider having an HIV test and thus be in a position to consider this opportunity for early treatment.

Asymptomatic stage

The asymptomatic stage of HIV-associated illness can last for many years. Although you may feel healthy during this time, the blood test for the HIV antibody is positive and, in most people who are left untreated, symptomatic disease and AIDS will develop.

Sometimes, swollen lymph nodes or glands may develop; this is called persistent generalised lymphadenopathy (or PGL) and is not a sign of damage in itself.

Symptomatic phase

As the infected immune system becomes more and more damaged, it is likely that the individual will either experience non-specific symptoms or become prone to infections that are likely to be the result of the impaired immunity, for example, fever, diarrhoea or weight loss. It is important that these are investigated to exclude any more serious underlying problem that needs treating (aside from HIV).

Infections that may occur during this phase include:

◆ candida (or thrush) in the mouth or throat; this fungal infection usually causes an odd taste and looks like white patches in the mouth;

◆ oral hairy leukoplakia, a viral infection that causes white patches along the side of the tongue; and

◆ shingles can occur in people with normal immune systems, but this condition occurs more often and more severely in those with HIV, causing blistering and a painful rash, which may be found across different parts of the body.

AIDS

Someone with HIV is said to have developed AIDS when one or more specific conditions are diagnosed. These can be summarised as:

◆ infections that would not cause the same illness in a person with an intact immune system (opportunistic infections);

◆ tumours or cancers that are unusual in a person with an intact immune system but are more frequently seen in those infected with HIV; and

◆ diseases that are a direct result of the infection, including dementia and 'wasting syndrome' (marked weight loss with diarrhoea and fevers without other cause).

Remember that the term 'AIDS' is an artificial one, drawn up by scientists trying to understand HIV infection and how it affects people. Different countries may have slightly different definitions of what constitutes AIDS and these may vary over time. Several years ago, it was thought that a diagnosis of 'AIDS' would help to predict how long the patient might live. However, newer treatments for both HIV and its complications have made the use of the term questionable. Some AIDS conditions are now relatively straightforward to treat and can be followed by prolonged good health whereas others still carry a poor outlook. Any individual may experience a different pattern of illness to any other, and in some people multiple illnesses occur or are recognised at the same time.

Opportunistic infections

These infections are of four major types:

◆ fungal;
◆ bacterial;
◆ protozoal; and
◆ viral.

Fungal infections

These include thrush or candidiasis, which can involve the mouth in symptomatic infection and can spread to the gullet (or oesophagus) in someone with AIDS, causing difficulty in swallowing.

Pneumocystis carinii is a fungus that causes a type of pneumonia, known as *Pneumocystis carinii* pneumonia (PCP). Symptoms associated with PCP occur gradually, with increasing breathlessness, dry cough and fever.

Cryptococcus can cause pneumonia and meningitis (inflammation of the lining of the brain). High fever and headache may develop and, in severe cases, the patient may become increasingly drowsy and confused.

Histoplasmosis infection is not seen commonly in HIV-infected patients in the United Kingdom, but is common worldwide. It can recur years after the initial infection and cause pneumonia or bone marrow infection with fever, anaemia and, occasionally, a rash.

Bacterial infections

Infection with the bacterium *Mycobacterium tuberculosis* causes tuberculosis (TB). This is usually isolated in the lungs, where it causes a chronic cough with sputum, associated with fever, night sweats and weight loss. In the context of HIV infection, it is not unusual for other parts of the body to be affected, as well as or instead of the lungs. Rarely (in the United Kingdom), TB may be resistant to many of the treatments available (multidrug-resistant TB) and require complex antibiotic therapy and prolonged isolation in special facilities.

Other types of mycobacterial infection are widespread in nature and largely pose a problem for individuals with severely weakened immune systems. These bacteria can spread throughout the body and are found in the blood, the bone marrow and the liver. *Mycobacterium avium–intracellulare* (MAI), also known as *Mycobacterium avium* complex (MAC), is the most common and causes fever, weight loss and anaemia.

Infection with the bacterium *Salmonella* causes diarrhoea in many people, but can cause severe and recurrent disease in those infected with HIV.

Protozoal infections

Protozoa are parasitic infections that can recur years after the initial infection and cause problems.

Toxoplasma can infect anyone who eats poorly cooked meat or comes in contact with infected cat excreta. The infection can reactivate in people with damaged immune systems and can form abscesses or pockets of infection in the brain. In severe cases, this can mimic a stroke or cause a fit.

Cryptosporidial infection can cause diarrhoea in anyone, but this can be very severe in an HIV-infected individual and can be difficult to clear; this may result in dehydration and nutritional problems.

Viral infections

Infection with a member of the herpes virus family called cytomegalovirus (CMV) is common in the general population. In people with very severe immune system damage, the virus can reactivate and cause retinitis (inflammation of the back of the eye), which can cause visual blurring or the sudden appearance of blobs that appear to float in front of the eye (floaters). CMV can also cause disease in the gut and the nervous system.

A virus called the JC virus (not the same virus as that associated with bovine spongiform encephalopathy or BSE) can produce abnormal areas in the brain called progressive multifocal leucoencephalopathy (PML), which may appear like a stroke.

Tumours

The two most common types of tumours occurring in HIV-infected patients are Kaposi's sarcoma (KS) and lymphoma.

Kaposi's sarcoma is a form of cancer that can affect the skin or internal organs of people infected with HIV. It develops as a growth of cells in blood vessel walls and is thought to be due to infection with a virus called human herpesvirus 8. It is usually seen as a thickened red or purplish lump on the skin or mouth; multiple lesions (damaged areas) often occur at the same time at different sites. It is rarely painful, but can cause a distressing cosmetic problem for some, and can follow an aggressive course in which lesions are found internally, affecting the lungs and gut.

Lymphoma is a tumour of the lymph tissues. It can develop anywhere in the body, including the brain. It is a serious illness, which may be difficult to diagnose, and non-specific features such as fever and weight loss are often present. Other symptoms vary according to the site of the tumour. Lymphoma may be one of the few HIV-related illnesses that has not been reduced by the use of newer anti-HIV therapies.

Why do some people become unwell sooner than others?

It is well known that some people become unwell sooner than others, although the reasons why are often not understood. Much current research is aimed at a better understanding of this variation, in the hope that this may help to suggest future treatment approaches. The possible reasons include:

◆ some people are not known to be infected with HIV until many years after the infection occurred and may, indeed, be unwell at the time of diagnosis;

◆ some people have taken anti-HIV therapies early enough to prevent or delay the onset of illness;

◆ some people have immune systems that are better than others at controlling the rate of HIV production and can maintain a stronger immune system for longer;

◆ some people may have genetic differences that give them a higher or lower risk of immune damage from HIV;

◆ some people may be infected by different types of virus; and

◆ some people may have other lifestyle factors that may make them more or less at risk of immune damage from HIV.

Since these reasons are poorly understood, it is often very difficult to provide accurate predictions about what may happen to any particular person.

6 Laboratory tests and monitoring

Clinic visits

Most people with HIV infection are under the medical supervision of a specialist clinic. Here, the doctors and other healthcare workers are familiar with the issues facing people living with HIV, the use and interpretation of new laboratory tests and the rapidly changing developments in the treatment of HIV.

It is usual for doctor and patient to establish a long-term partnership, in which each understands and respects the other's views and treatment decisions are made together. Any new tests or new drugs are discussed and you are encouraged to gain an understanding of your own particular illness and how to interpret any new changes.

Regular appointments are usually planned at least 3 monthly, with reviews of recent blood tests (see below) and a discussion of any new issues that have arisen since the previous visit. If you have recently begun therapy or your disease has laboratory features or a clinical picture that is more complex than usual, visits may be arranged at much shorter intervals. Similarly, if you notice any new or alarming symptoms, you should attend as soon as possible or discuss the problem with one of the healthcare team.

Symptoms that should raise concern include:

◆ unexplained weight loss;
◆ fever;
◆ breathlessness;
◆ diarrhoea;
◆ visual disturbance;
◆ headache;
◆ fits or leg/arm weakness; and
◆ unusual skin rashes.

Blood tests

Many different types of blood tests are performed at each regular review or if your condition suggests that a test may be necessary. Some of the more common tests are described here.

A full blood count will show how well your bone marrow is working and ensures that you are not low in red blood cells (anaemic), white blood cells (prone to infection) or platelets (prone to bleeding). Renal and liver function tests are performed to make sure that your liver and kidneys are working normally.

In addition, different tests may be performed to ensure that any drug therapy is not causing harm, for example blood fat levels or amylase (pancreas blood test).

Shortly after diagnosis, blood tests are usually performed to establish which other infections you may have been exposed to, so that any future risks may be minimised or appropriate measures taken. These would usually include tests for hepatitis (A, B and C), syphilis, toxoplasmosis and CMV.

CD4 counts

CD4 T-cell counts are blood tests that measure the number of these cells in a specimen of blood. The counts are used to estimate how well your immune system is functioning at the time of the test and this helps to determine whether you may be at risk of HIV-related complications.

CD4 counts only measure the number of CD4 cells in the blood (although most are found in lymph nodes and body organs). Moreover, these counts are influenced by sex (women tend to have higher CD4 counts), age (children have higher CD4 counts), smoking (smokers have higher counts) and other variables such as exercise and sleep.

Nonetheless, blood CD4 measurements appear to be fairly good predictors of the infections or tumours to which an HIV-infected individual may be prone (Figure 5).

Over time, in the absence of anti-HIV therapy, the CD4 count of an HIV-infected person will usually fall. The level to which it drops and the rate at which this happens are considered indications of the need for specific anti-HIV therapy or therapies, in order to prevent complications before they arise.

However, this is a matter for discussion between you and your doctor. Conversely, if you are already taking anti-HIV therapy, a rise in the CD4 count may be considered a marker of success.

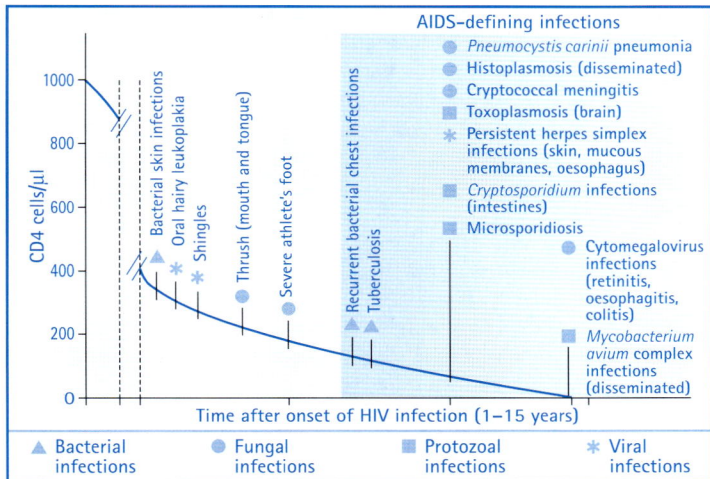

Figure 5: Graph of CD4 count over time, demonstrating levels at which the risk of illness becomes significant.

In a person without HIV infection, the CD4 count is usually in the range 400–1600 cells/μl. It is unusual to see HIV-related complications in anyone with a CD4 count higher than 350 cells/μl, and most AIDS-related illnesses occur in those with a CD4 count of 200 cells/μl or lower.

Viral load

Viral load tests use modern genetic techniques to measure the amount of the virus in a sample of blood. These measurements can be used in several ways:

◆ To predict how likely it is that the infected person will become unwell in the future.

◆ To provide extra information over and above the CD4 count in estimating the risk of becoming ill, especially if you are not already taking anti-HIV therapy. Put simply, a CD4 count tells you where you are, whereas a viral load test tells you where you are going. The higher the viral load, the higher the rate of new HIV particle formation, and the greater the risk that the immune system will be damaged more quickly.

◆ To assess how well anti-HIV treatment is working and to decide whether a change in treatment may be necessary.

One of the aims of treatment is to reduce the viral load as far as possible. In many people, if treatment is working well, the viral load will fall so far that it can no longer be measured using the currently available tests, and is considered 'below the limits of detection' or 'undetectable'. Nevertheless, small quantities of the virus will still be present in the blood, and probably larger quantities elsewhere in the body. Even if your viral load is 'undetectable', you may be able to infect others.

If you are taking anti-HIV treatment and your viral load is increasing, this suggests that HIV is increasingly able to form new particles. Therefore, it may be advisable to change to different drugs. Remember that your viral load will also increase if you stop taking your treatment or only take it from time to time. You must tell your doctor if this is the case, so that unnecessary, and possibly adverse, changes to treatment are not made.

Viral load tests can be performed by different methods. Therefore, moving to a new clinic where a different test is used may cause a change in your viral load. Currently, the tests are far from perfect, and if the same sample of blood is tested twice, it can give very different readings. Other infections or vaccinations might also cause the viral load to increase. It may be better to wait for a few weeks if this is the case, rather than having a viral load test that may be falsely high.

Other tests

Resistance tests

HIV can adapt to many of the drugs that are currently available for treatment, thus developing a certain amount of resistance. Sometimes, a blood test for drug resistance can indicate which drugs have stopped working because the virus has developed resistance. This information may help the infected person and the doctor to decide which drugs to use next. These tests are relatively new and may be used more often in the future when it is better understood how helpful they are.

Drug levels

Some people are better at absorbing drugs than others when taking the same number of tablets. It may be possible to measure how much drug is in the bloodstream and therefore to work out how much drug is needed. Again, these are very new tests and may be used more often when they are better understood.

7 Treatment of HIV

The treatments available to an HIV-infected patient can be broadly divided into two main types:

◆ Treatment for HIV itself
◆ Treatment for complications of HIV (see Chapter 8)

In the past few years, the number of drugs available to treat HIV has increased considerably (and will continue to do so). At the same time, knowledge of how best to use these drugs has improved, though many questions remain to be answered.

Although the currently available drugs do not provide a cure, they do reduce the likelihood that a person infected with HIV will become unwell from the complications of HIV, at least for several years. The widespread use of these drugs has caused a dramatic reduction in death rates and new cases of AIDS in all countries in which they are widely used.

Antiretroviral therapy

The drugs used to treat HIV are generally termed 'antiretrovirals', because they may also act against other members of the retrovirus family to which HIV belongs.

It is very clear the use of more than one drug at a time has better and longer-lasting effects than using one drug alone, and most people starting therapy today will take three or more drugs at once, called 'combination therapy'.

At present, there are three main types of drug, two types that act against the HIV reverse transcriptase enzyme and a third type that acts against the HIV protease enzyme (see Figure 2, page 5).

Nucleoside analogue reverse transcriptase inhibitors ('nukes' or NRTIs) mimic the building blocks of DNA and RNA and block this HIV enzyme by preventing new building blocks from joining the DNA chain.

Non-nucleoside reverse transcriptase inhibitors ('non-nukes' or NNRTIs) directly inhibit the reverse transcriptase enzyme.

Protease inhibitors block the protease enzyme (see Figure 2) and so prevent new forms of the virus from maturing and infecting other cells.

Most combination therapies use two NRTIs plus either an NNRTI or a protease inhibitor, or sometimes three NRTIs. People who have been treated already but need a new combination may be given a different mix of classes and/or more than three drugs. The currently licensed drugs are listed in Table 1.

Newer drugs are becoming available and this list may not be comprehensive.

Table 1: Currently licensed drugs for HIV therapy

Nucleoside analogue reverse transcriptase inhibitors

◆ AZT or ZDV (zidovudine; Retrovir®)
◆ ddC (zalcitabine; Hivid®)
◆ ddI (didanosine; Videx®)
◆ 3TC (lamivudine; Epivir®)
◆ d4T (stavudine; Zerit®)
◆ Abacavir (Ziagen®)

Non-nucleoside reverse transcriptase inhibitors

◆ Nevirapine (Viramune®)
◆ Efavirenz (Sustiva®)

Protease inhibitors

◆ Saquinavir (Invirase® or Fortovase®)
◆ Indinavir (Crixivan®)
◆ Ritonavir (Norvir®)
◆ Nelfinavir (Viracept®)
◆ Amprenavir (Agenerase®)

The aim of treatment

The aim of treatment is, ultimately, to improve the quality and quantity of life in an individual with HIV infection. Under certain circumstances, however, there are other, over-riding aims, such as post-exposure prophylaxis (see Chapter 3) and treatment of pregnant women (see Chapter 10).

It is believed that the best way to provide a longer lifespan and better life for people living with HIV is to reduce the viral load (quantity of virus in the blood) to as low a level as possible for as long as possible. This should help to prevent the virus causing further damage to the immune system and, hopefully, allow the immune system to recover some of the function it may have lost. Most people who are treated do, indeed, show an increasing CD4 count during treatment.

When to take treatment

There are many different opinions on the best time to start antiretroviral therapy. National and international committees meet regularly to discuss this question (among others). The decision will usually be taken between patient and doctor, based upon four issues:

◆ The clinical status of the patient: have there been any HIV-related illnesses to suggest that the immune system is already severely damaged?

◆ The CD4 count: is there a risk of the patient becoming unwell at the moment?

◆ The viral load: is there a risk of the patient becoming unwell in the near future?

◆ The patient: is he/she ready to start taking medications on a regular basis for the foreseeable future?

Taking medicines regularly

Taking antiretroviral therapy should, at present, be viewed as a long-term commitment. Drugs must be taken in the quantities prescribed, in the way recommended (for example, with or without food) and at the recommended times. If doses are missed or not enough drug is in the bloodstream, the virus can adapt and become resistant to one or more of the drugs in a combination. This can result in the viral load increasing and the combination no longer working. Subsequent combinations may be less effective if resistance has developed.

It is very important, therefore, to get things right from the beginning. It is best not to rush into taking antiretroviral therapy if possible, but rather to discuss plans for a new daily routine with your doctor, pharmacist or nurse before you take any action. If you are having problems with your planned routine, you should let your doctor know as soon as possible, so that alternatives can be considered.

Side effects

Like any other medications, antiretroviral drugs can cause side effects. These commonly occur in the first few weeks of treatment and may only last a short period of time (for example, sickness and headaches); simple drugs may help to reduce these. Other side effects may last much longer (for example, diarrhoea) and require further medications to help control them.

Some side effects, such as severe rashes or neuropathy (burning pains or 'pins and needles' in the feet and hands), may be so bad that you have to stop taking the drug. Since some of these drugs have been used only for a relatively short period of time (e.g. several years), long-term side effects are not fully understood. Many people who have been taking combination therapy for over a year have noticed that their body fat is wasting away in certain areas (upper arms and legs) and increasing in others (stomach and breasts). This effect, termed 'lipodystrophy', has yet to be fully explained.

If you develop symptoms which may be due to side effects of any antiretroviral therapy that you are taking, tell your doctor first, before you stop taking the drug. If the side effect is very severe, seek advice immediately. It is important not to adjust the dose or to stop taking medication without advice.

Drug interactions

Many drugs can interfere with the way that the body handles other drugs. For example, drug levels may be increased (with a risk of side effects) or decreased (with a risk of treatment failure and resistance) by interactions with other drugs. This is particularly the case for protease inhibitors and NNRTIs. Pharmacists and doctors will warn you about major interactions but you need to be careful about any other drug you are taking at the same time as the anti-HIV therapy, even drugs that can be bought over the counter (such as antihistamines, herbal remedies or recreational drugs). If you are any doubt, consult your pharmacist.

Changing or stopping treatment

There are situations where it may be necessary to change or to stop taking drugs that treat HIV. These include:

◆ when the treatment is no longer working (if the viral load is increasing or the CD4 count is decreasing);

◆ when side effects are not manageable; and

◆ when the daily routine is too difficult to manage.

In these, or any other, situations always seek advice before stopping one or all of the drugs so that the best treatment decision can be made.

8 Treatment of HIV complications and other therapies

Preventing complications

Some of the illnesses that used to be common in people with HIV are less likely today if preventative medicines are taken.

If you have never had an illness but may be at risk of developing it (usually based on the CD4 count), treatment may be recommended to reduce the chances of becoming unwell; this is called primary prophylaxis.

If you have had an HIV-related illness and there is a risk that it might return, treatment may be recommended to reduce this likelihood; this is called secondary prophylaxis.

Not all of these HIV-related infections can be completely cured. Therefore, after an episode of illness and appropriate treatment, lower doses may be used to prevent relapse; this is called suppressive or maintenance therapy. For example, when the CD4 count falls below 200 cells/µl, PCP may develop (see Opportunistic infections in Chapter 5). With a CD4 count at this level, primary prophylaxis against PCP is usually recommended to reduce the chance of it developing. For those HIV-infected patients who suffered from PCP previously and were healed after successful treatment, secondary prophylaxis may be recommended to reduce the risk of it developing again.

Primary prophylaxis against MAI and toxoplasmosis (see Opportunistic infections in Chapter 5) may also be considered. Infection with CMV at the back of the eye can be treated, but maintenance therapy is usually required to prevent it from relapsing.

For many people, the best way of preventing HIV complications may be to improve the immune function, using anti-HIV therapy. If you have begun therapy after having been unwell or having had a low CD4 count, it is not clear whether you can safely discontinue prophylaxis or maintenance therapy and you should discuss this with your doctor.

Treating complications

There are many treatments available for the range of infections and tumours that can occur in association with HIV infection and many complications respond well to treatment.

The first step is to make a correct diagnosis. This may involve a period of hospitalisation for investigations and initial treatment although, in some cases, outpatient management or day-case attendance may be possible.

The types of investigation that will be recommended depend on your symptoms and on what diagnosis is suspected.

If the problem is believed to be in the chest, a bronchoscopy may be required. This involves passing a tube through the nostrils or mouth and into the airways so that the lungs can be examined.

If the problem is believed to be in the gut, an endoscopy (passing a tube through the mouth and into the stomach) or a colonoscopy (passing a tube through the rectum and into the colon) may be required.

If there appears to be a nervous system disorder, a scan of the brain and/or an analysis of fluid from the spine (lumbar puncture) may be needed.

Treatment will be directed towards the proven diagnosis, or the most likely diagnosis if you are unwell or it is difficult to make a definite diagnosis. You should discuss the treatment options with your doctor, who will provide more detailed information.

Generally, anti-infective drugs will be used for proven or suspected infections. In many circumstances, these will require intravenous administration of drugs followed by a course of tablets or capsules. In some cases, there may be no tablet preparation available and a prolonged course of intravenous therapy may be required. For some serious infections (e.g. CMV), intravenous therapy may be required at intervals for the rest of your life. For a few infections, no proven treatment option is available.

Your chances of responding successfully to treatment for an infection will be increased by improving your immune function. Therefore, anti-HIV therapy may be discussed and usually started at this point.

Treatment of tumours associated with HIV can be managed in several ways. Chemotherapy with intravenous and/or oral drug regimens are often used. In some circumstances, X-ray treatment (radiotherapy) may be the best option, but sometimes (particularly with early Kaposi's sarcoma), a watch-and-see approach may be best.

Involvement of the patient in treatment decisions

Today, the medical and allied professions recognise that you must be able to make your own decisions about your treatment in conjunction with your doctor. This recognition is probably best seen in the care of people with HIV, largely because people infected with or affected by HIV have made great contributions to our current understanding of the illness and how to treat it.

You should be given as much information and support as possible to enable you to make a decision that is in your own best interests. There are times when patients decide to withdraw from the aggressive management of complications, for which treatment options may be limited, and to concentrate on controlling symptoms and maintaining a certain quality of life rather than prolonging life. All people with HIV should be able to discuss their wishes with their healthcare team.

Complementary therapies

The therapeutic effects of diet, minerals, vitamins and homeopathy remain under investigation. Although there are many claims of immune-boosting effects for these approaches, they have not yet been subject to the same level of scientific testing as antiretroviral or anti-infective agents. For many people, these are seen as complementary rather than alternatives to conventional therapeutic approaches. However, you should be cautious about using any of these alternative therapies. Some vitamins or minerals can be toxic if used excessively, changes in diet can lead to deficiencies in nutrients and any substance may have a potential for interactions with prescribed treatments.

Other therapies, including massage, aromatherapy, reflexology and acupuncture can be very helpful to those infected with HIV. They can help not only with stress, but also to treat specific symptoms and to ease some of the side effects associated with prescribed medicines.

With many questions about the best treatment approaches remaining unanswered and with many new drugs in the pipeline, HIV-infected patients, particularly those attending larger treatment centres, may well be asked to participate in a clinical trial.

Trials are performed to show whether a new treatment or new way of using an existing treatment is as good as or better than conventional therapies.

Trials can be designed in many different ways. In most cases there is a 'control arm', a group of people receiving standard or current best therapy, and a 'treatment arm', a group of people receiving the treatment under investigation. Usually, people entering the trial will not be allowed to choose which group to join, but are selected for one or the other at random by computer. In some trials, placebos or dummy drugs are used so that neither the patient nor the doctor knows which type of treatment is being used for that individual.

All clinical trials are planned thoroughly, with patient safety in mind, and will have been approved by an Ethics Committee, who are responsible for protecting the rights of patients in the trial.

Before anyone is invited to enter a trial, the doctor will have assessed that person to determine whether the trial may be beneficial. The trial will also have typical characteristics, which the potential patient must fulfil (inclusion criteria), and safety criteria, which the potential patient must not have (exclusion criteria). If all these criteria are met, and you are invited, then you must consider whether it is in your interests to take part. Common reasons why people do or do not want to take part in trials are listed in Table 2 (see page 40).

If you are unsure about entering a clinical trial, the doctor or research nurse can provide more information and will be happy to discuss it further. Remember: it is your decision whether to enter or not, and if you choose not to enter, your medical care will not otherwise be affected. Moreover, if this is not the right time to enter a trial, there will probably be other trials in the future.

Table 2: Advantages and disadvantages of entering clinical trials

Advantages

◆ Access to new drugs
◆ More frequent monitoring
◆ Most up-to-date monitoring techniques
◆ Benefit to others

Disadvantages

◆ More frequent clinic visits
◆ Placebo may be unacceptable
◆ May involve too many tablets
◆ Anxieties about unknown side effects

10 Women and HIV

Epidemiology

Globally, the most important route of HIV transmission is through heterosexual intercourse and men and women are infected in equal numbers. Within the UK, the number of people newly diagnosed with HIV infection each year has stayed much the same for the last 10 years. However, the number of people who have become infected through heterosexual intercourse has been increasing rapidly and now one-third of all infections in the UK occur through heterosexual intercourse. There has been a parallel rise in the number of children infected through mother-to-child transmission. Surveys of women attending antenatal clinics in London indicate that, in some hospitals, 1 in 200 pregnant women is HIV-positive, but most of these women are unaware that they are infected. With the recent advances in HIV treatment, most cases of AIDS in the UK also occur among men and women unaware that they are HIV-positive. This is particularly true for men and women who have acquired HIV through heterosexual intercourse.

Risk factors for heterosexual transmission of HIV

The risk of HIV infection during a single episode of heterosexual intercourse with an HIV-positive partner is approximately 1 in 300. One important risk factor is the amount of infectious virus in the blood (or viral load) of the infectious partner, which is high shortly after first infection and also late in the course of the infection. This pattern of viral load can result in the rapid spread of HIV to multiple concurrent sexual partners early in infection. Later, the risk of infection risk is lower, which partly explains why some couples in stable relationships may be 'discordant' for HIV, that is, one partner remains uninfected despite unprotected sexual intercourse with the HIV-positive partner over a long period of time. The use of condoms protects both partners against HIV transmission and this is very important, because the risk of transmission is always present and may increase again with time. In one study in Europe, no transmission of HIV occurred between 'discordant' couples who always used condoms.

The presence of infections of the genital tract also increases the risk of HIV transmission, by increasing the infectiousness of the HIV-positive partner and by increasing the susceptibility of the uninfected partner. This applies both to infections that are sexually transmitted, such as gonorrhoea, chlamydia and genital ulcers, and to infections that are not sexually transmitted, such as candida and bacterial vaginosis (BV). Vaginal candida and BV are the most common causes of vaginal discharge.

Family planning

From time to time there has been concern about whether contraception (other than condoms) may increase the risk of HIV transmission. Intrauterine devices (IUDs) have been associated with an increased risk of pelvic infection shortly after insertion, but this can be avoided by appropriate screening for asymptomatic infection or prophylactic antibiotics. IUDs do not provide protection against HIV transmission. Moreover, oral contraceptive pills and long-acting (depot) intramuscular injections of progesterone are more reliable contraceptives than standard IUDs.

The more recently developed progesterone-releasing IUD (mirena) is more effective than standard IUDs and has additional advantages, since it may improve any dysmenorrhoea (also known as menorrhalgia) and the risk of pelvic infection is smaller. The main disadvantage is that an initial change in the pattern and duration of menses is common, with spotting or prolonged bleeding. There has been concern that depot injections may increase susceptibility to HIV by thinning the vaginal mucosa. However, a recent study of women attending a family planning clinic in Dar es Salaam showed that none of these three contraceptive methods was associated with an increased risk of HIV infection. For women who have completed their families, tubal ligation is the most efficient contraception, and it is irreversible. The regular use of condoms in addition to these more efficient methods of contraception is recommended to protect both partners against HIV and other sexually transmitted infections.

Fertility

Although untreated sexually transmitted infections, such as chlamydia, may reduce the chances of subsequent conception, because of damage to the fallopian tubes, HIV infection itself does not have any effect on fertility. It has been suggested that women diagnosed with HIV are more likely to have had an earlier miscarriage, sometimes so early that the woman does not realise that she has ever been pregnant. Even in non-HIV-infected women, approximately 30% of conceptions are 'lost' in this way.

Gynaecology

Although a decrease in levels of testosterone, the 'male' sex hormone, can occur in HIV infection, production of the 'female' sex hormones, oestrogen and progesterone, is normal in otherwise well HIV-infected women. Menstruation is not affected by HIV infection.

Abnormal cervical or pap smears are more common in HIV-infected women, and annual smear tests are recommended rather than tests every 3 years. Colposcopy, which allows a more detailed visual examination of the cervix with light and magnification, is better than a routine smear, as any abnormal areas of the cervix can be more easily recognised and biopsied. Cervical carcinoma was added to the list of AIDS-defining illnesses in the 1993 because, sometimes, the abnormal cells seen on pap smears become cancerous. However, most abnormal smears are due to mild abnormalities that can improve without treatment. Sometimes, the abnormal cells must be treated to prevent a cancer developing. Cervical cancer is a very uncommon AIDS-defining illness, and some studies suggest that it occurs no more frequently in HIV-infected than non-HIV-infected women. Nearly all cases of cervical cancer result from infection of the cervix with a subtype of human papillomavirus (HPV). The use of condoms helps protect women against this infection.

Vaginal candida and genital ulcers due to the herpes simplex virus often recur and are more likely to do so in women with HIV infection. Both conditions occur while the immune system is still relatively strong and do not mean that you have AIDS. Both conditions are treatable. If either develops very frequently, you can take a drug regularly to prevent new episodes.

Pregnancy

Without intervention, the risk of mother-to-child transmission of HIV has been up to 25% in Europe and nearer 50% in developing countries. Approximately one-half of all transmissions occur at the time the child is born and one-third are due to breast-feeding. Only one-sixth of infections occur before delivery and nearly all occur in the last few weeks of pregnancy. It is rare for the foetus to become infected with HIV during the first 6 months of pregnancy. With appropriate care and education of the expectant mother, 99% of babies born to HIV-infected women will not be infected with HIV (see section on Drug treatment for mother and baby, below). Further risk will be prevented if the baby is not breast-fed.

The risk of transmission of HIV is not the same for all women. The viral load is very important, and high viral loads are associated with transmission rates above 50% if untreated. Low CD4 cell counts and the clinical stage of HIV in the mother (symptomatic or with AIDS) are also helpful in predicting the risk of transmission. A low risk of transmission is seen in women with low viral loads but, at present, there appears to be no threshold of viral load below which transmission does not occur.

Caesarian section reduces the risk of infection by at least 50%, but only if performed before labour begins. This is known as an elective Caesarian section.

Drug treatment for mother and baby

If the antiretroviral drug zidovudine (known as AZT or ZDV) is taken by the mother before and during labour and by the baby for up to the first 6 weeks of life, the risk of transmission is reduced by two-thirds. Shorter courses of AZT (starting at week 36 of the pregnancy) have reduced transmission by one-half. In two studies in Europe, the risk of HIV transmission to babies who were formula-fed, whose mothers had an elective Caesarian section and also took AZT, was less than 1 in 100. New studies with the drug nevirapine suggest that a single dose taken by the mother at the onset of labour and a single dose taken by the baby at 24–72 hours of age provide more protection than a very short course of AZT.

Although the safety of AZT (or nevirapine) in pregnancy is not proven, many thousands of women and their babies have now taken AZT safely. Rare complications of therapy cannot be ruled out, but the benefits far outweigh any risk. Fewer data are available for other antiretroviral therapies. In the interests of both mother and child, these therapies are usually started, with caution, in the second and third trimesters of pregnancy unless the mother requires earlier treatment for her own health.

Planning a pregnancy while on antiretroviral therapy

Recently, the number of women conceiving who are already on antiretroviral therapy has increased quite dramatically. Usually, by the time the mother has realised that she is pregnant and discussed this with her doctor, the embryo has already been exposed to a number of medications for several weeks. In these circumstances, the advantages of continuing with treatment often outweigh the potential risk of the baby being born with a deformity. At present, no-one knows what effects these treatments for the mother have on the unborn child, nor how safe they are, particularly during the first 3 months of pregnancy. Other commonly prescribed treatments, such as co-trimoxazole or dapsone and pyrimethamine for PCP prophylaxis, may also cause congenital abnormalities. Therefore, if you are taking treatment for HIV and you are considering having a baby, you should discuss the situation with your doctor first. It may be worth taking 400 mg folic acid daily if you plan to become pregnant.

HIV testing in antenatal clinics

If you are pregnant and you do not know you are HIV-positive, HIV infection of the baby cannot be prevented. Therefore, when you attend an antenatal clinic, you will be strongly advised to have an HIV test.

If you are HIV-positive, pregnancy itself will not have an adverse effect on your health. However, premature delivery (before week 37) is more common in women with HIV infection, particularly those with more advanced disease. Premature labour is also associated with a higher risk of mother-to-child transmission. For these reasons, antiretroviral therapy to prevent mother-to-child transmission is commonly started at weeks 29–32 of pregnancy. Longer courses of antiretroviral therapy do not appear to be necessary and may allow AZT-resistant virus to emerge. However, in a recent study, in which mothers started AZT monotherapy as early as the start of week 14, AZT resistance was uncommon.

Current guidelines for HIV-infected pregnant women

Current guidelines suggest that, for women who would not normally be offered antiretroviral therapy, the combination of formula-feeding rather than breast-feeding, elective Caesarian section and a short course of AZT is appropriate to protect the baby.

For women with more advanced HIV infection, in whom treatment with antiretroviral therapy would be recommended if they were not pregnant, triple antiretroviral therapy should be commenced after the first 3 months of pregnancy. This will suppress HIV replication and reduce the risk of transmission as well as allowing the immune system to recover. At present (until more data are available), an elective Caesarian section should be considered and all babies should be formula-fed.

11 Children and HIV

HIV infection affects not only an individual patient but also entire families. Therefore, all children with HIV infection must be seen as part of a family.

Routes of transmission

Mother–to–child transmission
Children infected with HIV usually acquire the virus from their mothers (see Chapter 10). Most are infected around the time of birth, although transmission can occur earlier in pregnancy. Infection may also occur after birth if an infected mother breast-feeds her baby.

Blood products
With routine screening of blood products in the UK, this is no longer regarded as a route of transmission. However, some HIV-infected children may have acquired the infection from blood products in other areas of the world where donated blood is not routinely screened.

Sexual transmission
Occasionally, boys and girls acquire the infection through consenting or non-consenting sexual activity. The numbers, however, remain low.

Diagnosis

All babies born to HIV-infected women will have maternal HIV antibodies in their blood, which usually disappear by the age of 18 months. In the past, it has been difficult to test children between birth and 18 months of age. However, in recent years, a technique known as polymerase chain reaction (PCR) has allowed a diagnosis by 4 months of age in most cases.

After the age of 18 months, a positive HIV antibody test will confirm that an infant has HIV infection.

In addition to blood testing, assessment of a child's clinical condition may suggest the presence of HIV infection. Signs and symptoms can include delayed physical development, enlargement of the lymph glands and certain organs (e.g. liver and spleen), inflammation of the parotid glands, persistent oral candidiasis (thrush), recurrent chest or ear infections, chronic or recurrent diarrhoea and poor weight gain. None of these signs and symptoms occur only with HIV infection and a confirmatory blood test must be done. In some cases, a mother may not realise she has HIV infection until her baby develops a severe infection.

Immunisation

For HIV-positive children, routine immunisations are recommended, with certain alterations. Live vaccines are avoided where possible and, therefore, inactivated (injectable) poliomyelitis (polio) vaccine is recommended in place of oral polio drops. The use of Bacille Calmette–Guérin (BCG) vaccine is not recommended because of the risk of dissemination. Immunoglobulin may be used in children after exposure to measles and varicella zoster (chickenpox), although each child is assessed according to existing immune function and previous exposure to these viruses.

Table 3 contains the current recommended immunisation schedule for HIV-infected children.

Family–based care

With differing cultures, what may be good healthcare practice in one population may be inappropriate or impractical in another. Wherever possible, parents and their HIV-infected children should attend the HIV clinic together. Family-based care should be a universal goal where HIV-infected children are concerned, especially when more than one family member is infected. This type of care will not only give better support to the infected child (and any other infected family members) but also help the family as a whole to cope with the infection. There is also evidence that this approach reduces distress and disturbance among the other, uninfected children of the family.

Treatment

While most treatments used for adults are available for children, there are special concerns when treating children, both social and medical. In this respect, children cannot simply be regarded as diminutive adults. If you have an HIV-infected child you must think

Table 3: Schedule of vaccination for the immunisation of HIV-infected children
Bacille Calmette–Guérin (BCG)
Not recommended
Hepatitis B
Birth, then at 1, 2 and 12 months
Diphtheria, tetanus and pertussis (DTP), *Haemophilus influenzae* **B (HIB) and meningococcal C**
At 2, 3 and 4 months
Poliomyelitis (polio; inactivated vaccine)
At 2, 3 and 4 months
Measles, mumps and rubella (MMR)
At 12–15 months and preschool booster
Diphtheria and tetanus (DT) and polio (inactivated)
Preschool booster

carefully about the consequences for the child and for the whole family before deciding whether the child will be treated. Remember, once the virus is acquired, it will be in the body for life. Current therapy is unable to eliminate the virus.

Medical concerns

Drug distribution and metabolism within the body varies according to the growth and development of the child. This means that great care must be taken by the doctor when selecting dosages. The type of drug formulation given, whether oral liquid, tablets or injections, may also affect children to a greater extent than adults, especially if the drug has a particularly nasty taste, as many do.

Social factors

There will be a need to ensure that the child takes the required medicine, at the proper times. At what age should a child be told of the diagnosis? Some children cope better, both emotionally and physically, with the disease than others. Perhaps most important of all, it is clear that any form of treatment will affect the child's quality of life, and this must be taken into account when making treatment decisions. The adolescent, for example, is particularly concerned with body image, peer and parent relationships and independence.

Guidelines for therapy in HIV-infected children are currently based on informed opinion, rather than clear-cut evidence. Nevertheless, in infants under the age of 1 year, there are compelling arguments for aggressive intervention, although there may be difficulties with long-term tolerability and adherence.

It is unanimously agreed that, if well-tolerated, effective, safe anti-HIV combinations were available, all children should be treated as soon as they are diagnosed. This is not yet the case.

Schooling

HIV-infected children of school age do not pose a risk to other children. In the event of possible exposure to body fluids, standard precautions should be followed for all children without exception. Knowledge that a child is HIV-positive should not alter the management of the child or the situation.

If your child is diagnosed HIV-positive, you do not have to tell anyone at the school. However, if you want to tell someone at your child's school, it may be best to choose a permanent staff member with authority, such as a head-teacher. If someone within the school is aware of the diagnosis, he/she can tell you about the presence of infections such as measles or chickenpox, which might affect your child.

Nutrition

Children with HIV infection may occasionally suffer from gastro-intestinal disturbances, resulting in nutritional deficiencies, weight loss and 'failure to thrive'. Dietary assessments to ensure optimal nutritional intake are a routine part of a child's care.

Certain micro-organisms known as cryptosporidia may occasionally get into water supplies, causing diarrhoea in some people with weakened immune systems. Boiling all drinking water will ensure that these germs are killed.

12 General advice

Food and drink

Most people's diets include a suitable mixture of carbohydrates, protein, fat, minerals and vitamins. However, many of the illnesses associated with HIV can cause weight loss and many of the treatments for HIV may require a change in dietary habits. Therefore, if you are infected with HIV, you may need to seek help from time to time from a dietitian, who will ensure that you are meeting your dietary needs, particularly if you have lost weight.

Food poisoning, in particular, may have more serious consequences in people with damaged immune systems and, therefore, HIV-infected people should:

◆ avoid raw or under-cooked meats and eggs;
◆ avoid unpasteurised milk and cheese; and
◆ wash vegetables thoroughly.

Infections may also be picked up from contaminated water. In particular, the parasite *Cryptosporidium* can infect water and, in individuals with impaired immune systems, cause severe diarrhoea that can be difficult to treat. Bottled water may also be contaminated, and many water filters are not effective in removing the organism. Ideally, if you have a CD4 count of <200 cells/µl, you should boil all drinking water, cooling it for drinking if required.

Alcohol, in moderate amounts, is probably not harmful. Large quantities of alcohol may, however slow down recovery from infections, and can make it difficult to remember to take medications. Some medications react badly with alcohol, but this should be made clear at the time the treatment is dispensed.

Recreational drugs

There is no clear evidence that the immune system can be damaged by using recreational drugs. People who continue to share needles may be re-infected with HIV and will certainly be at risk of other blood infections. Stimulant drugs (such as ecstasy, amphetamines or cocaine) may interact with anti-HIV medications and if you use any of these substances, you should discuss the possible risks with your doctor. Poppers remain a source of controversy; many people have argued that they can impair the immune system, though the evidence for this is not clear-cut at all. Certainly, men who use the impotence drug sildenafil (Viagra) should not use poppers.

Travelling

If you are planning a holiday abroad and you are HIV-positive, it is worth checking whether there are any difficulties with entry into your country of destination. Some governments still impose barriers against people with HIV. The laws can change from time to time and the relevant embassy or high commission should be able to give you up-to-date information.

Travel insurance can be problematic for people with HIV. With one or two exceptions, policies will not cover medical expenses for HIV-related health issues. It is still worth taking insurance to cover lost property, cancellations, and non-HIV-related medical claims.

Most vaccinations required to travel are not a problem for a person with HIV, except for yellow fever vaccination, which you should avoid. Poliomyelitis (polio) vaccinations can be given as a live or dead vaccine, but the dead (inactivated) vaccine is safer for people with HIV.

Travelling while taking combination therapy can pose some difficulties. First, it is advisable to take a doctor's letter explaining what medications you will be bringing through customs, to show if you are questioned. Second, time-zone changes can cause disruptions in your routine. You should discuss the best way of preparing for this disruption with your doctor or pharmacist. Third, some medications may require special storage in hot countries or may need an increased fluid intake. Again, pharmacists can provide valuable advice.

General practitioners and dentists

Many people choose not to tell their general practitioners (GPs) of their HIV status, in case the information is disclosed to others, or do not use their GPs because of concerns about lack of experience in this area of medicine. Most HIV clinics, however, provide ongoing information to help GPs manage HIV-infected patients in partnership or 'shared care'. This may be particularly helpful if the patient lives a long way from the HIV clinic. Some GPs provide 24-hour medical cover and/or home visits, and most are likely to be more skilled than the HIV specialist with general health issues. If the HIV-infected patient finds it hard to obtain a suitable GP, help is usually available from either the local health authority or the HIV clinic.

If you decide not to tell your GP that you are HIV-positive, you should let your HIV clinic doctor know and, particularly if you are admitted to hospital, you should tell the ward doctor. Remember that commonly prescribed medicines can interact with anti-HIV medicines, so that if a GP prescribes medicines for a general health issue without knowing that you are taking other medications, you will need to check that there is no known risk involved.

Many people with HIV have difficulties with mouth and gum infections, and problems with their teeth. You should tell your dentist if you are HIV-positive, so that he can give you the most appropriate treatment. Although all dentists can provide dental care to people with HIV, some choose not to do so. If you have difficulty finding a dentist, your health authority or HIV clinic should be able to help.

Pets

Certain infections that can cause diseases in people with HIV can originate from pets. In many cases, however, these diseases represent reactivation of old infections rather than new infections. It is unlikely, therefore, that people with HIV will need to avoid pets that they have had for many years. Nevertheless, you should discuss this with your doctor. For example, it has been recommended that cat litter should be handled by others or with gloves, that animals should have annual veterinarian (vet) checks and be regularly treated for fleas.

13 Legal and financial issues

All HIV-infected individuals must consider the legal issues surrounding their condition. In any legal situation, whether you are HIV-infected or not, it is difficult to be sure of your rights. You should not be afraid to seek professional advice: everyone is entitled to legal advice and assistance.

Insurance

Many situations can arise in which your HIV status or sexuality may be requested for insurance purposes. This may occur when you apply for health or life insurance or for an endowment mortgage. Travel insurance may also be affected. An insurance company is not legally obliged to insure anyone and it does not have to give reasons for refusing your insurance. When you complete a 'proposal' or application form, you are under a duty to disclose anything that may be a 'material factor' affecting the insurance, whether you are asked about it or not. If the policy is issued and the insurance company finds out that you have not been honest, the policy is not valid and is made void.

To assess an application where health may be an issue, the insurance company will consider the information in your proposal form, which will include a medical questionnaire or report prepared by your doctor and, possibly, a supplementary questionnaire, for example a 'lifestyle' questionnaire, which will ask about your personal/social life.

Remember that the insurance company cannot ask for a medical report without your consent. Obviously, if you refuse, you will not be insured. You have the right to see your doctor's medical report about you before it is sent, but you may have to ask for it in writing. Ask the surgery for advice if you want to see your doctor's report and are unsure how to go about it. Many doctors refuse to answer the lifestyle questionnaire; it may be worth asking your GP what answers he/she would give if approached and discussing their usefulness.

An insurance company may ask you to visit your own doctor for a medical examination, for example if the company knows or suspects you are in one of the 'high-risk' groups, if you apply to be insured for a large sum of money or your doctor discloses anything in your past medical records that indicates a higher than average health risk. You have no right to see a medical report prepared by the insurance company's doctor.

Your proposal form is likely to be treated cautiously if you have been refused insurance before or have had particular terms imposed (such as a higher premium). If this is the case, you will already be on a national computer list. If you think you may be refused, you should withdraw your proposal in writing before it happens.

If you are HIV-negative, you should not be refused insurance solely because you have had an HIV test. If you took the test on your own initiative, they may consider this an indication of lifestyle and may either refuse insurance or offer it at a higher premium. Most insurance companies no longer ask about previous HIV tests, but only about positive tests or other sexually transmitted diseases.

If you are HIV-positive you will not get life insurance at this point in time. If you get health insurance, it will not cover HIV-related illnesses.

If you are gay or bisexual, your proposal will not be rejected outright by all companies. Some will consider you if you are in a stable relationship and test HIV-negative, although premiums may be higher.

Different companies take different views, and some companies take a more liberal stance than others. It is wise to seek advice from an independent financial advisor before deciding which company to ask for insurance.

The Association of British Insurers provides free advice on insurance matters (but will not recommend specific companies):

The Association of British Insurers, 51 Gresham Street, London EC2V 7HQ. Tel: 020 7600 3333.

Mortgages

Even if you cannot get life insurance, you may still be able to get a mortgage.

Some types of mortgages require life insurance, for example endowment, pension-linked and foreign currency mortgages. Lenders often want you to take out a new life insurance policy for the mortgage, because they are paid commission by the life insurance company.

If you are likely to be refused life insurance, you can apply for a repayment mortgage or an interest-only mortgage. The lender may insist on life insurance if you are borrowing a large amount of money, if the value of the property is similar to the amount you wish to borrow or if you are seeking a mortgage protection policy. In this type of situation, independent financial advisors should be able to give you good advice.

Problems in the workplace

With the exception of medical and allied professionals, nobody has ever been shown to have been infected with HIV through their work duties. However, cases of discrimination have been recognised for many years. While there is no specific employment law for people infected with HIV, government guidance and the Disability Discrimination Act (1996) provide some protection. The guidance suggests that all employers should have a policy for dealing with employees who have HIV infection or AIDS. People who are asymptomatic, while not directly protected by any legislation, should (according to government guidance) be treated no differently from other employees.

HIV tests

Some employers insist on their employees having an HIV test. There is no law to prevent this, but you cannot be forced to have a test against your will. The employer does not have the right to know the result but can refuse to employ you if you do not disclose the result or if it is positive.

If you have already had a positive HIV test, your doctor cannot inform an employer of the result without your permission, unless it is considered to be in the public interest. Your doctor owes a duty of confidentiality to you as a patient. If your employer knows that you have the virus, that information is strictly confidential and must not be passed on to anyone else without your permission. The major exception to this, where disclosure is considered to be in the public interest, is for healthcare workers who perform exposure-prone procedures (predominantly surgeons).

Symptomatic infection or AIDS

People with symptomatic infection or AIDS should be protected under the Disability Discrimination Act. Under this law, if you have symptomatic HIV, you should not be treated less favourably than any one else, unless there is good reason. This applies to recruitment, training, promotion and dismissal. Employers are expected to make reasonable adjustments to the workplace to allow HIV-infected people to perform their duties, and are unable to reject an applicant outright purely on the basis of a previous HIV-related illness.

There is no requirement to allow more sick leave for HIV-infected employees than for any other employee, although some companies have developed policies that specifically acknowledge the pattern of illness associated with HIV to enable HIV-positive employees to remain in work. If an HIV-infected employee becomes ill, the employer should consider all the circumstances, including the individual's ability to do the job, the possibility of a transfer to different duties and any medical advice from, if possible, an occupational physician. The HIV-infected employee should be treated in exactly the same way as an employee with any other non-contagious life-threatening illness. Under employment protection legislation, an employee who has been dismissed but has been with the employer for 2 years or more has the right to take a case to an industrial tribunal on the grounds that the dismissal was unfair. The qualifying periods are 2 years of continuous employment for those employed to work more than 16 hours a week, and 5 years of continuous employment for those employed to work less than 16 but at least 8 hours per week.

Special precautions are not needed in most workplaces. Healthcare workers need to take normal protective measures to avoid direct contact with blood and other body fluids. Similar procedures should also apply to those who may be accidentally exposed to body fluids or discarded needles (for example, those in community work and emergency services). Guidance is available from Health Departments.

Hygiene precautions should always be taken to reduce the risk of any infection, including HIV. You should wear protective gloves to clean up any blood or body-fluid spillage when giving anyone first aid and wash your hands thoroughly afterwards.

Financial support

Although there is no state benefit support specifically targeting people with HIV, there are a large number of benefits for which an HIV-infected person may be eligible. These may apply to people who are in or out of work, and people who are seeking employment or unable to work because of poor health. There are also various personal schemes and both national and local charitable organisations to which you can apply.

Since any application will be dependent on individual factors, local factors and changes in the benefit system, people infected or affected by HIV should seek advice from their local Benefits Agency or HIV/AIDS agencies.

14 The future

S ome of the most important questions for the future are:

◆ Will HIV continue to spread and cause a high level of mortality?
◆ When will a successful vaccine be developed to prevent infection with HIV?
◆ When will there be a cure for HIV disease?

Will HIV continue to cause a high level of mortality?

The simple and sad answer to this is yes, the HIV epidemic will continue to spread and cause a high level of mortality. However, in the developed world and where individuals can afford it, highly active antiretroviral therapy (HAART) has had a major impact on mortality rates, especially in the United Kingdom, Western Europe and the United States. Hence, in the United Kingdom, for example, the number of new cases of full-blown AIDS occurring each year is decreasing. However, given the uncertainties of the long-term benefits and difficulties with these medications, and the large number of people who are not yet aware of their HIV status, this picture may change.

Most cases of HIV/AIDS are in sub-Saharan Africa, which has close to 70% of the global total of HIV-positive people, followed by Asia and Latin America, in countries where poverty and poor health systems allow very limited resources for prevention and care. Thus, 90% of the world's HIV-infected people have no access to antiretroviral therapy. Most of these will die in the next 10 years. It is therefore essential that Western societies help to promote HIV/AIDS education and support in less well-developed countries while continuing to provide health education about HIV to the populations of their own countries.

Can a successful vaccine be developed to prevent infection with HIV?

As yet, no successful vaccine has been developed and there are still many years of research ahead before this can happen. One of the greatest difficulties is that there are so many subtypes of HIV. Therefore, it is difficult to provide protection against all the different strains of HIV to which an individual might become exposed. Optimists predict that a good vaccine may be available within 5 years, whereas pessimists say that it seems unlikely at present that a vaccine will ever become possible.

Wherever the truth lies, research progress is still being made and large amounts of funds are still forthcoming for this purpose.

Will there be a cure for HIV disease?

The best treatments currently available for HIV merely slow down the growth of the virus although, in some selected patients, HIV growth may almost reach a standstill. While many new treatments are being developed, it is premature to suggest that we are close to a cure. With currently available treatment options, it is still thought to be impossible to eliminate the virus from an HIV-infected person.

15 Answers to questions you may be asking yourself

I can't make up my mind whether to have an HIV test. What should I do?

This is discussed in detail in Chapter 4. Most clinics have specially trained advisors or counsellors who will discuss the pros and cons of having a test with you and will help you to make a decision.

Why do some people get AIDS quickly and others not?

This is not understood fully. Some people show very rapid progression and others show slow progression or even no progression at all (these are known as long-term non-progressors). It may be that some viral strains are more virulent than others or, perhaps, certain people have immune factors that make it possible to withstand the virus. Long-term non-progressors are being studied carefully to see if light can be shed on this phenomenon.

Does everybody with HIV get AIDS?

We do not know. It may be that long-term non-progressors will never develop AIDS or that new treatments may maintain the immune system for many years; only time and experience will tell.

How long do most people with AIDS live?

No-one can say for certain, especially if the patient is properly treated with modern drugs, because some people respond better than others. Ten years ago the average survival of a patient with AIDS was only 6 months, then it became 2–3 years and now it may be up to 10 years. Survival is likely to depend on the particular 'AIDS' condition that a patient has: some are more easily treated than others.

How safe is a blood transfusion nowadays?

Blood transfusion is very safe in most industrialised countries as potential donors from high-risk groups are discouraged from donating and all blood is screened. In less affluent countries, the screening tests may not be available and it is a good general principle not to agree to a blood transfusion unless it is absolutely necessary.

My son attends the same school as another child who is said to have HIV infection. What should I do? What should I tell him?

The only risk to your son would be if he had a major playground fight with his HIV-infected friend. Rather than making a special fuss, you should teach your son to be careful with any blood spillages whatever the source and to report any incidents to the teachers, who are trained to deal with any situation that may be considered a 'high-risk' event.

My daughter was playing in the park and was pricked by some used needles which appear to have been left by drug users. What should I do?

Wash the area of skin thoroughly and report to your general practitioner or Casualty Department. There is a higher risk of hepatitis infections than of other viruses in this setting and a course of vaccinations may be recommended. The risk of HIV transmission is very small; however, your general practitioner can advise and arrange blood tests as necessary.

If I am diagnosed as having HIV, how often will I need to go to hospital?

Most people with HIV choose to attend a specialist HIV clinic regularly, both to monitor their health and to discuss treatments and new advances in the area of HIV medicine. Those who have no symptoms and have CD4 counts above 500 cells/μl and a low viral load may be seen every 4–6 months. Those with more advanced infection or on complex treatments may be seen at least every 6 weeks.

Staff at a typical clinic will discuss any symptoms and psychological well-being as well as blood testing for CD4 cells, viral load measurements and, occasionally, measurements of liver and kidney functions. Doctors will also check for swollen glands and any other changes in physical health.

Most large clinics provide a variety of support services, including specialist nurses, pharmacists, counsellors, health advisors, psychologist and dieticians, to give additional advice and support. Furthermore, clinics frequently have links with complementary therapists who are able to provide massage, aromatherapy and acupuncture as well as other therapies.

Should I tell my general practitioner if I am HIV positive?

Ideally, you should tell your general practitioner. The specialist HIV clinic that you attend will then keep your general practitioner informed of your progress, who may also help from time to time. If you would rather not involve your general practitioner, then perhaps you should think about changing to another practice. If you still decide not to involve your general practitioner at all, then you should tell your clinic, so that they do not send the general practitioner correspondence related to your condition.

Should I tell my dentist if I am HIV positive?

You should let your dentist know, ideally. If he/she is aware of your HIV status, the dentist can also check for any complications that can affect the mouth.

I am pregnant and have tested positive for HIV infection. What should I do?

Discuss the situation with your obstetrician. Great progress has been made in recent years in preventing the transmission of HIV from mother to child. Using anti-HIV therapies and avoiding breast-feeding, will significantly reduce the chances of transmission. Your obstetrician and/or HIV doctor will be able to guide you through the latest information.

Is oral sex safe?

Oral sex carries some risks. It is advisable to avoid ejaculation in the mouth and to avoid oral sex if there are cuts and sores present. Some people choose to use condoms for oral sex to be even safer.

My doctor tells me my viral load is undetectable. Can I stop taking my drugs?

If your viral load is 'undetectable', this only means that current blood tests cannot measure the virus. There will still be virus elsewhere in the body, and you will still be HIV antibody positive. If you stop taking your drugs, it is likely that the viral load will rise rapidly (although, in a few people worldwide, this has not been the case). It is recommended that you discuss *any* change to your drug routine with your doctor before doing it.

If I discover I am HIV positive should I contact all recent sexual partners?

The decision of whom to tell can be difficult. The counsellor or doctor who gives you your result should advise you on questions like this. It may be helpful for your contacts to know that they may be at risk of infection or may already be HIV positive without being aware of this.

I keep forgetting to take doses on time. What should I do?

The first thing you must do is immediately tell the doctor who prescribed the medicine for you. There is a great danger that you may be ruining the effect of the drug. You and your doctor together should decide what is the best thing to do.

I have been told that some herbal medicines, including cannabis, are useful in treating HIV. Is this true?

Herbal medicines, including cannabis, have been used widely by people living with HIV. They have not been shown to be beneficial in treating HIV itself, but many people report that they can be helpful in managing symptoms or side effects. It is important, however, to ensure that they are safe to take with prescribed medicines (as some changes have been reported) and to discuss these issues with your doctor or pharmacist.

What about ecstasy or 'harder' drugs?

There has been at least one death reported as due to an interaction between ecstasy and the anti-HIV drug ritonavir. Other anti-HIV drugs may also evoke reactions with recreational drugs. Very little knowledge is available in this area and the risk cannot be assessed accurately. It is wise to discuss your use of recreational drugs with your doctor in order to be fully aware of the potential risks.

16 Support groups

If you have HIV or AIDS, or you are worried about these diseases, it is important that you know you are not alone. Many patients find it useful and comforting to share their experiences with others in the same situation. For this reason, there are support groups, advice services and self-help groups throughout the United Kingdom and in most major towns and cities all over the world. There are also many local groups, and information should be available from doctors' surgeries or from directories at local libraries. Moreover, do not forget the support that certain church communities may be able to give.

Most large hospitals will have a patient support group. Often, such groups will put out a newsletter or organise talks by specialists or professional carers working in the field. This is also a good way of learning about new treatment advances.

The following national and international associations will give emotional support and practical help to men and women infected with HIV and to their families, friends and carers. The addresses given are often for a head office and there may be many branch offices. A freephone number can often be used to gain information about groups in your area.

This is not an exhaustive list. In particular, the websites listed for these organisations frequently point the user towards other helpful organisations supplying additional specialist information on treatment, symptoms, patient support groups and recent research findings.

United Kingdom

ACIA

ACIA is a voluntary organisation which offers buddying, support group meetings and other services for Africans living with HIV/AIDS.

African Community Involvement Association

Eagle Court, 224 London Road, Mitcham CR4 3HD
Tel: 020 8687 2400

Fax: 020 8646 4363
(mobile: 0956 988 481)
Website: http://www.tht.org.uk/acia/aciaindx.htm

Africa Advocacy Foundation

HIV treatment information, advocacy and education for people living with HIV/AIDS their family and carers, particularly those from sub-Saharan Africa.

Africa Advocacy Foundation

4 Crowndale Centre,
218 Eversholt Street, London NW1 1BD
Tel: 020 7691 0234
Fax: 020 7691 0222

AIDS AHEAD (AIDS Health Education & Advice for the Deaf)

AIDS AHEAD

17 Macon Court, Herald Drive,
Crewe CW1 6EE
Tel: 01270 250 736 (voice)
text: 01270 250 743
Helpline: 01270 250 743 (Wed 7–10pm)
Minicom: 01606 47736 (Bulletin Board)
Fax: 01270 250 742

aidsmap

A website produced by the National AIDS manual in conjunction with the British HIV Association

aidsmap

Website: http://www.aidsmap.com

AIDS Treatment Project (ATP)

HIV/AIDS treatment education and advocacy from a HIV positive-led membership-based group.

AIDS Treatment Project (ATP)

St Stephen's House,
115-129 Southwark Bridge Road,
London SE1 0AX
Tel: 020 7407 0777
Helpline: 0645 470047 (Mon & Wed 6–9pm)
Fax: 020 7403 4262
Email: admin@atp.org.uk
Website: http://www.atp.org.uk

AVERT

This charity aims to prevent people becoming infected with HIV, to work towards a cure and to improve the quality of life of those already infected.

AVERT

4 Brighton Road, Horsham, RH13 5BA
Tel: 01403 210 202
Fax: 01403 211 001
Email: avert@dial.pipex.com
Website: http://www.avert.org/

Blackliners

A national telephone helpline for people affected by HIV/AIDS who are of African, Caribbean or Asian descent.

Blackliners

Unit 46, Eurolink Centre, 49 Effra Road, London SW2 1BZ
Tel: 020 7738 7468 (admin)
Helpline: 020 7738 5274 (Mon–Fri 10–6.30pm)
Fax: 020 7738 7945
Email: bliners@aol.com

Body & Soul

A self-help organisation supporting women, heterosexual men, their children and families living with or affected by HIV/AIDS.

Body & Soul

The Royal Homoeopathic Hospital,
60 Great Ormond Street, London WC1N 3HR
Tel: 020 7833 4828 (admin)
Tel: 020 7833 4929 (client line)
Fax: 020 7833 4898
Email: info@bodyandsoul. demon.co.uk
Website: httm://www.bodyandsoul.demon.co.uk

British Medical Association Foundation For AIDS

British Medical Association Foundation For AIDS

BMA House, Tavistock Square, London WC1H 9JP
Tel: 020 7383 6315 (admin)
Helpline: 020 7383 6345 (Mon–Fri 9–5pm, professional enquiries only)
Fax: 020 7388 2544
Email: aidsfdn@bmaids.demon.co.uk
Website: http://www.bmaids.demon.co.uk

Continuum

A pro-life organisation for long-term survivors and for those who wish to remain healthy after an HIV or AIDS diagnosis.

Continuum

172 Foundling Court, Brunswick Centre,
London WC1N 1QE
Tel: 020 7713 7071 (admin)
Fax: 020 7713 7072
Email: continu@dircon.co.uk
Website: http://www.users.dircon.co.uk/~continu/

Children with AIDS Charity

Supporting families affected or infected with HIV or AIDS.

Children with AIDS Charity (CWAC)

2nd Floor, 111 High Holborn, London, WC1V 6JS
Tel: 020 7242 3883
Fax: 020 7242 3884
Website: http://www.cwac.org

Crusaid

CRUSAID is the leading fund-raising charity for AIDS relief in the UK. It is dedicated to maintaining the dignity and improving the quality of life for people with HIV.

Crusaid

73 Collier Street, London N1 9BE
Tel: 020 7833 3939 (admin)
Tel: 020 7833 9707 (hardship fund)
Fax: 020 7833 8644
Email: office@crusaid.org.uk

DHIVA (Dietitians in HIV/AIDS Group)

DHIVA is a recognised group of the British Dietetic Association (BDA) consisting of dietitians who specialise in working with people with HIV infection or who have an interest in the area of nutrition and HIV infection.

DHIVA

Dept of Nutrition & Dietetics,
Royal Free Hospital Trust,
Pond Street,
London NW3 2QG
Tel: 020 7830 2056
Fax: 020 7830 2251

Edward King's AIDS pages

A wide range of overviews of key topics in HIV treatment and prevention, each packed with links to the best sources of online information.

Edward King's AIDS pages

Website: http://www.users.dircon.co.uk/~eking/index.htm

The Eileen Trust

This is a charitable trust, funded by the Government, which exists to help people who were infected with HIV as a result of treatment within the NHS involving whole blood transfusion, tissue transplant or blood products (but not including people with haemophilia, whom the Macfarlane Trust exists to help).

The Eileen Trust

Alliance House,
12 Caxton Street,
London SW1H 0QS
Tel: 020 7799 3184 (admin)
Helpline: 020 7799 3184 (Mon–Fri 9.15–5pm)
Fax: 020 7233 0839

Elton John AIDS Foundation

The Foundation is an international non-profit organisation providing funding for services which alleviate the physical, emotional and financial hardship caused by HIV/AIDS, as well as prevention education projects.

Elton John AIDS Foundation

1 Blythe Street, London W14 0HG
Tel: 020 7603 9996
Fax: 020 7348 4848

European Forum on HIV/AIDS Children & Families

The European Forum has been established to promote the needs of children and families affected by HIV in Europe.

European Forum on HIV/AIDS Children & Families

c/o London Lighthouse,
111–117 Lancaster Road,
London W11 1QT
Tel: 020 8383 5697
Fax: 020 8383 5620
Email: naomi@euskida.demon.co.uk

Europoz

For positive people in the UK and Europe. Europoz is an electronic mailing list for people who are HIV positive in Europe. It is intended to be a supportive forum where people of any gender and sexuality can exchange information and experiences relating to HIV and AIDS issues.

Europoz

Website: http://www.diversity.org.uk

FACTS (Foundation For AIDS Counselling Treatment & Support)

FACTS provides specialised in-practice training and education to GPs and other healthcare workers. General training courses are designed for other groups, home care workers, teachers etc. Support and advice is available to professional staff.

FACTS

FACTS Centre,
23-25 Weston Park,
London N8 9SY
Tel: 020 8348 9195
Fax: 020 8340 5864

Gay Men Fighting AIDS (GMFA)

Gay Men Fighting AIDS

Unit 42,
Eurolink Centre,
49 Effra Road,
London SW2 1BZ
Tel: 020 7738 6872
Fax: 020 7738 7140
Email: gmfa@gmfa.demon.co.uk
Website: http://www.demon.co.uk/gmfa

The Georgehousetrust

Supports people affected by HIV in the North West of England and campaigns for the best quality of life for all people with HIV.

The Georgehousetrust

77 Ardwick Green North
Manchester M12 6FX
Tel: 0161 274 4499
Fax: 0161 274 3355
Website: http://www.georgehousetrust.org.uk/

Get Wired

HIV treatment information. How to get started and where to look.

Get Wired

Website:
http://www.getwired.co.uk/en/1/currentissue_5.html

The Haemophilia Society

The Haemophilia Society

Chesterfield House,
385 Euston Road,
London NW1 3AU
Tel: 020 7380 0600
Fax: 020 7387 8220
Email: info@haemophilia-soc.demon.co.uk
Website: http://www.haemophilia-soc.demon.co.uk

Health & Housing

Information, news, training and projects. Supported accommodation for people with AIDS and HIV.

Health & Housing

Room 65,
London Fruit Exchange,
1 Brushfield Street,
London E1 6EP
Tel: 020 7375 3553
Fax: 020 7375 0577
Email: info@healthhousing.org.uk
Website: http://www.vois.org.uk/healthhousing/

HIV Care

A treatment information website run by Glaxo Wellcome for patients and health professionals.

HIV Care

Website: http://www.hivcare.co.uk/

Hospice Information Service

Hospice Information Service

St Christopher's Hospice,
51–59 Lawrie Park Road,
London SE2 6DZ
Tel: 020 8778 9252 x262/263
Fax: 020 8776 9345

Immune Development Trust

A clinic offering a broad range of holistic therapies to people living with HIV.

Immune Development Trust

90–92 Islington High Street,
London N1 8EG
Tel: 020 7704 1555 (admin)
Tel: 020 7704 1777 (client line)
Fax: 020 7226 9001

International Community of Women Living With HIV/AIDS

International Community of Women Living With HIV/AIDS

2c Leroy House, 436 Essex Road,
London N1 3QP
Tel: 020 7704 0606
Fax: 020 7704 8070
Email: icw@gn.apc.org
Website: http://www.icw.org

Jewish AIDS Trust

Established to provide the Jewish community with education, counselling and support in connection with HIV infection and AIDS.

Jewish AIDS Trust

Colindale Hospital, Colindale Avenue,
London NW9 5HG
Tel: 020 8200 0369
Fax: 020 8200 1345
Email: jat@ort.org
Website: http://www.jat.ort.org

Lesbian & Gay Bereavement Project

Lesbian & Gay Bereavement Project offers telephone support, advice and counselling to lesbians and gay men bereaved by the death of a partner or otherwise affected by bereavement.

Lesbian & Gay Bereavement Project

Vaughan M Williams Centre,
Colindale Hospital, Colindale Avenue,
London NW9 5HG
Tel: 020 8200 0511 (admin)
Helpline: 020 8455 8894 (Mon–Sun 7pm–midnight)
Fax: 020 8200 1345
Email: lgbp@aol.com
Website: http://home.aol.com.lgbp

Macfarlane Trust

This trust provides advice and some funds to people with haemophilia who were infected with HIV as a result of treatment for haemophilia, their dependants and those who have died.

Macfarlane Trust

Alliance House, 12 Caxton Street,
London SW1H 0QS
Tel: 020 7233 0342 (admin)
Helpline: 020 7233 0342 (Mon–Fri 9.15–5pm)
Fax: 020 7233 0839

NAM Publications (National AIDS Manual)

NAM is the leading information provider on HIV and AIDS in the UK.

NAM Publications

16a Clapham Common Southside,
London SW4 7AB
Tel: 020 7627 3200 (admin)

Helpline: 020 7738 5274 (Mon–Fri 10–6.30)
Fax: 020 7627 3101
Email: info@nam.org.uk
Website: http://www.aidsmap.com

National AIDS Helpline

This is a 24-hour national phone line offering confidential counselling, advice, information and referrals on any aspect of HIV/AIDS to anyone.

National AIDS Helpline

PO Box 5000, Glasgow G12 8BR
Tel: 0141 357 1774 (admin)
Helpline: 0800 567123 (Mon–Sun 24hr)
Fax: 0141 334 0299
Minicom: 0800 521 361 (Mon–Sun 10–10pm)
Email: network@netscot.co.uk

National AIDS Trust (NAT)

The National AIDS Trust (NAT) campaigns to promote effective prevention, quality treatment and care, support for the development of vaccines and an end to discrimination against people with HIV/AIDS.

National AIDS Trust

New City Cloisters, 188–196 Old Street,
London EC1V 9FR
Tel: 020 7814 6767
Fax: 020 7216 0111
Email: info@nat.org.uk
Website: http://www.nat.org.uk/nat/

National HIV Nurses Association (NHIVNA)

National HIV Nurses Association

Organising Secretariat,
1 Mountview Court, 310 Friern Barnet Lane,
London N20 0LD
Tel: 01895 829207(admin)
Fax: 01895 820852
Email: kepple@pharmaresearch.com
http://www.soh.brad.ac.uk/hodgsi/nhivna/index/htm

National Long Term Survivors Group

The group offers support to men and women living with an HIV-positive diagnosis for five years or longer.

National Long Term Survivors Group

PO Box BMLTSG, London WC1X 3NN
Tel: 020 7735 9685
Fax: 020 7735 9685

The Naz Project London

The Naz Project is an HIV/AIDS education, prevention and support service for people within Greater London who are members of the South Asian, Middle Eastern and North African communities and communities from the Horn of Africa.

The Naz Project London

Palingswick House (Annexe),
241 King Street,
London W6 9LP
The entrance is situated off Weltji Road
Tel: 020 8741 1879 (admin)

Helpline: 020 8741 1879 (Mon–Fri 9.30–5.30pm)
Fax: 020 8741 9609
Email: nazlon@dircon.co.uk

The Network of Self-Help HIV and AIDS Groups

Aims to promote good networking between new and existing HIV self-help and support groups throughout the country.

The Network of Self Help HIV and AIDS Groups

4th Floor Sophia House,
23–35 Featherstone Street,
London EC1Y 8QX
Tel: 020 7250 1540
Fax: 020 7250 1560
Email: network@dircon.co.uk
Website: http://www.network.dircon.co.uk/

PACT (The Association of NHS Providers of AIDS Care & Treatment)

This national association is primarily concerned with advocacy for its members, especially around issues such as client confidentiality and contract funding applications.

PACT

c/o Andrewes Unit,
4th Floor KGV,
St Bartholomew's Hospital,
London EC1A 7BE
Tel: 020 7601 7847
Tel: 020 7601 8428
Fax: 020 7601 8057

Paediatric AIDS Resource Centre (PARC)

Information resources for individuals and organisations involved with children and families infected with or affected by HIV.

Paediatric AIDS Resource Centre

20 Sylvan Place,
Edinburgh EH9 1UW
Tel: 0131 536 0806 (admin)
Fax: 0131 536 0841
Email: ams@srv2.med.ed.ac.uk
Website: http://www.ed.ac.uk/~clah/parc.html

Positively Healthy (PH)

Positively Healthy is a long-established UK gay men's holistic HIV/AIDS charity, entirely operated and managed by its service users.

Positively Healthy

PO Box 71, Richmond-upon-Thames,
Surrey TW9 3DJ
Tel: 020 8977 4411
Fax: 020 8977 4411
Email: poshealth@declare.com

Positively Women

Positively Women was founded to provide a range of free and strictly confidential counselling and support services to women with AIDS and HIV.

Positively Women

347–349 City Road, London EC1V 1LR
Tel: 020 7713 0444 (admin)
Helpline: 020 7713 0222 (Mon Wed Thu Fri 10–4pm,
  Tue 10–2pm)
Fax: 020 7713 1020
Email: poswomen@dircon.co.uk

PPC (Positive Partners & Positively Children)

Provides both practical and emotional support to men, women and children affected by HIV/AIDS.

PPC

Unit F7, Shakespeare Commercial Centre,
245a Coldharbour Lane,
London SW9 8RR
Tel: 020 7738 7333 (admin)
Helpline: 020 7738 7399 (Wed 6–9.30pm)
Fax: 020 7501 9382

Red Ribbon International

A registered charity that has made the Red Ribbon into an internationally recognised symbol in the fight against AIDS.
Website: http://www.redrib.dircon.co.uk/

Sigma Research

Sigma Research is an independent research unit based in London but affiliated to the University of Portsmouth. It specialises in social and behavioural research into sexual behaviour, HIV and AIDS and related services.

Sigma Research

Unit 64 Eurolink Centre,
49 Effra Road,
London SW2 1BZ
Tel: 020 7737 6223
Email: admin@sigma-r.demon.co.uk
Fax: 020 7737 7898
http://www.sigma-r.demon.co.uk

Solas

A centre offering support services, information and informal meeting place for people living with HIV, HIV-related illnesses and with AIDS, their close family, partners and carers.

Solas

Support Centre,
2–4 Abbeymount,
Edinburgh EH8 8EJ
Tel: 0131 661 0982
Fax: 0131 652 1780
Email: mail@solas.semon.co.uk
Website: http://www.solas.demon.co.uk
Opening times: Mon, Tue, Thu, Fri 10–4pm, Wed 5–9pm.

The Sussex Beacon

A continuing care centre for people with HIV/AIDS related illnesses.

The Sussex Beacon

Bevendean Road,
Brighton, BN2 4DE
Tel: 01273 694 222
Fax: 01273 682 740
Website: http://www.pavilion.co.uk/beacon/contact.htm

The Terrence Higgins Trust (THT)

One of the first national voluntary organisations to respond to all aspects of the HIV/AIDS health crisis, this trust provides services to improve the health and quality of life of those affected and campaigns for greater public understanding.

The Terrence Higgins Trust

52–54 Grays Inn Road,
London WC1X 8JU
Tel: 020 7831 0330 (admin)
Helpline: 020 7242 1010 (Mon–Sun noon–10pm)
Fax: 020 7242 0121
Email: info@tht.org.uk
Website: http://www.tht.org.uk

Ugandan AIDS Action Fund (UAAF)

Assistance and advocacy for Africans affected by HIV/AIDS.

Ugandan AIDS Action Fund

Unit 333,
Great Guildford Business Square,
30 Great Guildford Street,
London SE1 0HS
Tel: 020 7928 3275 (admin)
Helpline: 020 7928 9583 (Mon–Fri 9–5pm)

The UK Coalition of People Living With HIV & AIDS Ltd

This national organisation of individuals living with HIV/AIDS provides user-led needs assessment services, consultancy, research and training on user involvement.

The UK Coalition of People Living With HIV & AIDS Ltd

250 Kennington Lane,
London SE11 5RD
Tel: 020 7564 2180 (general enquiries)
Fax: 020 7564 2140
Email: post@ukcoalition.demon.co.uk
Website: http://www.aids-advocacy.org

Vanguard AIDS Information Service

A charity providing HIV information and education services to the African refugee communities in London.

Vanguard AIDS Information Service

26b Thames House,
South Bank Commercial Centre,
140 Battersea Park Road,
London SW11 4NB
Tel: 020 7627 5170
Fax: 020 7622 7516
Email: vanguard@dircon.co.uk

UK treatment publications

AIDS Newsletter

A monthly newsletter summarising news on all AIDS issues including treatment developments.

AIDS Newsletter
CAB International, Wallingford,
Oxon, OX10 8DE
Tel: 01491 832111
Fax: 01491 833508

ATP Doctor Fax

A fortnightly compilation of research abstracts and conference reports collated from the Internet with commentary, aimed at doctors treating people with HIV.

ATP Doctor Fax
AIDS Treatment Project, St Stephen's House,
115–129 Southwark Bridge Road,
London SE1 0AX
Tel: 020 7407 0777
Email: admin@atp.org.uk

AIDS Treatment Update

A IDS Treatment Update is the first and only specialist British treatment newsletter. It is available free of charge to any individual affected by HIV or AIDS.

AIDS Treatment Update
NAM Publications,
16a Clapham Common Southside,
London SW4 7AB
Tel: 020 7637 3200
Fax: 020 7627 3101
Email: atu@nam.org.uk

Axiom Magazine

M onthly health and lifestyle magazine for gay men with particular focus on HIV, distributed free through clinics, bars and clubs in London and the UK.

Axiom Magazine
73 Collier Street, London N1 9BE
Tel: 020 7833 3399
Fax: 020 7837 2707

Continuum

P ublishes articles on alternative views regarding AIDS.

Continuum
172 Foundling Court,
Brunswick Centre,
London WC1N 1QE
Tel: 020 7713 7071

Current AIDS Literature

A monthly annotated bibliography with commissioned editorial commentaries, aimed at healthcare professionals and researchers.

Current AIDS Literature
CAB International,
Wallingford,
Oxon OX10 8DE

HIV & AIDS Current Trends

T his is a quarterly newletter aimed at practising clinicians, which contains up-to-date information on new treatments.

HIV & AIDS Current Trends
Mediscript Ltd,
1 Mountview Court
310 Friern Barnet Lane,
London N20 0LD

Mainliners Newsletter

P ublished approximately monthly, this newsletter includes treatment information aimed at HIV-positive drug users or ex-users.

Mainliners Newsletter
205 Stockwell Road,
London SW9 9SL
Tel: 020 7737 7472

Positive Nation

M onthly news magazine for HIV-positive people distributed free through GUM clinics, service organisations, gay pubs and clubs.

Positive Nation
250 Kennington Lane,
London SE11 5RD
Tel: 020 7564 2121
Fax: 020 7564 2128
Website: http://www.positivenation.co.uk

Positive Times

A monthly newspaper produced for people living with HIV and AIDS.

Positive Times
Cedar House,
72 Holloway Road,
London N7 8NZ
Tel: 020 7296 6222
Fax: 020 7296 0026
Email: postimes@aol.com

+ve

A imed at people affected by HIV/AIDS, including family, friends and carers.

+ve
1 Pembroke Road,
Ruislip,
Middlesex HA4 8NQ
Tel: 01895 637 878
Fax: 01895 637 273
Email: andrewb@akitanet.co.uk
Website: http://www.howsthat.co.uk

International listings

The Global Network of People living with HIV/AIDS (GNP+)

GNP+ aims to improve the quality of life of people living with HIV/AIDS.

The Global Network of People living with HIV/AIDS (GNP+)

Central Secretariat,
P.O. Box 11726,
1001 GS Amsterdam,
Netherlands
Tel: +31 20 689 8218
Fax: +31 20 689 8059
Email: gnp@gn.apc.org

The International AIDS Society (IAS)

The International AIDS Society

IAS Secretariat, P.O. Box 5619, SE-11486 Stockholm,
Sweden
Tel: +46 8 459 6621
Fax: +46 8 662 6095
Email: ias@congrex.se
Website: http://www.ias.se

IAS Affiliated Societies

Some IAS Affliated Societies

Argentina:
Sociedad Argentina de Sida (SAS)
Att: Dr Sergio Lupo
Donato Alvarez 73,
piso 12º C (1406)
Buenos Aires
Argentina
Tel: +54 1 633 4354
Fax: +54 1 304 2386

Belgium:
European AIDS Clinical Society (E.A.C.S)
Att: Prof. N. Clumeck
Saint Pierre University Hospital
Rue Haute, 322 (PL5)
BE-1000 Brussels
Belgium
Tel: +32 2 535 4130
Fax: +32 2 539 3614

Greece:
Hellenic Association for the Study and Control of AIDS
Att: Dr. G. Papaevangelou
PO Box 140 85
GR-11521 Athens
Greece
Tel: +30 1 646 7473
Fax: +30 1 721 5082

Italy:
Associazione Nazionale per la Lotta Contro l'Aids (ANLAIDS)
Att: Prof. Fernando Aiuti
Via Barberini 3
IT-00187 Roma
Italy
Tel: +39 6 482 0999
Fax: +39 6 482 1077

Korea:
Korean Alliance to Defeat AIDS (KADA)
Att: Sang Eun Lee
Room 307
Semi B/D #57, 8ka Youngdungpo-dong
Youngdungpo-ku
Seoul 150-038
Korea
Tel: +82 2 636 8060
Fax: +82 2 636 1526

Malaysia:
Malaysian Society for HIV Medicine
Att. Rokiah Ismail
c/o Dept. of Medicine
University of Malaya
50603 Kuala Lumpur
Malaysia
tel/Fax: +60 3 440 2351

Spain:
Sociedad Espanola Interdisciplinaria del SIDA (SEISIDA)
Att: Prof. Rafael Nájera
Bravo Murillo, 377 5oD
Apartado de Correos 42137
ES-28080 Madrid
Spain
Tel: +34 1 314 24 61
Fax: +34 1 314 35 96

The International Community of Women living with HIV/AIDS

This network of HIV-positive women has regional representatives in five global areas: Africa, Europe, North America, Latin America & the Caribbean and Southeast Asia & the Pacific. For UK details, see page 70.

The International Council of AIDS Service Organisations

The International Council of AIDS Service Organisations

ICASO Central Secretariat
399 Church Street
Toronto, Ontario,
Canada, M5B 2J6
Tel: +1 416 340 2437
Fax: +1 416 340 8224
Email: icaso@web.net
Website: http://www.web-net/~icaso/icaso.html

The Joint United Nations Programme on HIV/AIDS

The Joint United National Programme on HIV/AIDS

UNAIDS
20, avenue Appia
CH-1211 Geneva 27
Switzerland
Tel: +41 22 791 3666
Fax: +41 22 791 4187
Email: unaids@unaids.org
Website: http://www.unaids.org

Acquired immune deficiency syndrome (AIDS)
A diagnosis made when someone with HIV experiences specific infections or tumours regarded as a result of damage to the person's immune system. The term 'AIDS' may not necessarily be a useful indicator of future outlook, since the ability to treat different conditions varies greatly.

Acupuncture
An alternative therapy using needles inserted into various parts of the body.

Acute
A condition that develops rapidly.

Anaemia
A reduction in the number of red blood cells.

Anal sex
Sexual intercourse involving insertion of the penis into the anus or back passage.

Antibodies
Proteins in the body that help fight diseases. Antibodies are formed in response to infection with, for example, a virus or bacterium. If an individual is believed to be infected with a virus or bacterium, a test showing the presence of antibodies against that particular virus or bacterium will confirm that the person is infected.

Antiretrovirals
Drugs that are active against the retrovirus family to which HIV belongs.

Aromatherapy
An alternative treatment that uses aromatic plant extracts and oils.

Asymptomatic
Having no symptoms of a particular disease.

B lymphocytes
A group of cells that form part of the immune system. These cells are responsible for the formation of antibodies.

Bronchoscope
An instrument by which the inside of the tubes leading from throat to the lungs can be examined.

Candidiasis
An infection in which the fungus *Candida albicans* invades the linings of the body, for example the mouth or the vagina (thrush).

Cervical cap
See diaphragm.

Cervical secretion
Secretion from the neck of the womb.

Cervical (pap) smears
A test in which samples of cells are taken from the neck of the womb (cervix) to detect the presence of abnormal cells.

Chemotherapy
Treatment using chemical drugs (usually against tumours).

Chickenpox
An infection caused by the varicella zoster virus, which causes a painful, blistery rash.

Chromosomes
The genetic material that is present in every cell.

Colonoscopy
The use of a fibre-optic telescope on the end of flexible tube to examine the large bowel.

Colposcopy
The examination of the vagina and neck of the uterus using an instrument called a colposcope.

Cryptococcus
A yeast-like fungus that can cause pneumonia and meningitis.

Cryptosporidial infection
An infection caused by the parasite *Cryptosporidium parvum* which results in diarrhoea.

Cytomegalovirus (CMV)
A herpes virus that can cause damage to the back of the eye (retina), the bowel or other parts of the body in people with very damaged immune systems.

Dementia
Decreased concentration and rapidity of thought, loss of interest and slowness of physical movement.

Diaphragm
A contraceptive method in which a piece of rubber with a flexible rim fits in the vagina over the neck of the womb (cervix).

Diarrhoea
Frequent passing of unusually loose bowel movements.

DNA
Deoxyribonucleic acid, the genetic material of most living organisms, which controls heredity and is located in the cell nucleus.

Dysmenorrhoea
Pain occurring in the back or lower abdomen of a woman at the time of her monthly period (menses).

Endoscopy
A flexible tube that is passed into the body in to order to examine various parts.

Enzyme
A protein that speeds up reactions in the body.

Epidemic
A disease that has affected a large number of people in a particular area during a given time period.

Epstein–Barr virus
A virus of the herpes family that causes glandular fever (mononucleosis).

Factor VIII
A protein that is essential for blood clotting. It is absent in haemophiliacs.

Glandular fever
A disease caused by the Epstein–Barr virus, which affects the lymph glands and causes fever and sore throat. It is also known as mononucleosis.

Haemophilia
A hereditary bleeding disease caused by the deficiency or absence of Factor VIII in the blood, resulting in an inability to clot blood.

Hepatitis
Inflammation of the liver, which can be caused by infections or drugs.

Herpes simplex virus
A virus of the herpes family, which causes cold sores and genital herpes.

Histoplasmosis
A fungus that causes pneumonia, bone marrow infection with fever and, occasionally, rash.

Homeopathy
A form of alternative medicine using minute doses of drugs that, in a healthy person, would mimic the disease being treated.

Host cell
Cell acting as a host, in which HIV has become integrated into the chromosome and will remain there for the life of the cell.

Human immunodeficiency virus (HIV)
The virus that causes AIDS.

Immunoglobulin
A type of blood protein that functions as an antibody.

Intrauterine device (IUD or IUCD)
A small contraceptive device inserted into the uterus (womb).

Kaposi's sarcoma
A form of cancer that can affect the skin or internal organs. It is caused by a growth of cells in blood vessel walls and usually appears as a thickened red or purplish lump on the skin or mouth.

Leukoplakia
A viral infection that causes white patches along the side of the tongue.

Lipodystrophy
A disease, not very clearly defined, that may be caused by certain antiretroviral drugs. Body fat may be lost from some areas (upper arms and legs) and increased in others (stomach and breasts).

Lumbar puncture
The withdrawal of spinal fluid from the lower back with a hollow needle, usually for diagnosis.

Lymph, lymph nodes, lymphatic system, lymph vessels
Lymph is a colourless fluid containing white blood cells, proteins and fats. It is carried around the body in a network of minute vessels or tubes called the lymphatic system. Lymph nodes are small organs lying at quite frequent intervals along the course of a lymph vessel. They can act as a barrier to the spread of infection by destroying or filtering out bacteria or other agents.

Lymphoma
A general term relating to tumours arising from the cells of the lymph tissues.

Meningitis
Inflammation of the lining of the brain.

Menses
Monthly discharge of blood from the womb.

Mycobacterium avium complex (MAC)
A complex of two organisms, *Mycobacterium avium* and *Mycobacterium intracellulare*. Infection with these bacteria causes fever, weight loss and anaemia. This complex is also known as *Mycobacterium avium–intracellulare* (MAI).

Mycobacterium tuberculosis
A bacterium that causes tuberculosis.

Neuropathy
A disease of the nerves, which may be felt as burning pains or 'pins and needles' in the hands or feet.

Non-nucleoside reverse transcriptase inhibitors (NNRTIs)
These drugs directly inhibit the HIV enzyme reverse transcriptase.

Nonoxynol-9
A spermicidal agent contained in many spermicidal preparations.

Nucleoside reverse transcriptase inhibitors (NRTIs)
This class of anti-HIV drugs mimic the building blocks of DNA and RNA and acts against the HIV reverse transcriptase enzyme by preventing new building blocks from joining the DNA chain.

Opportunistic infection
An infection caused by bacteria, viruses or fungi that take the 'opportunity' to infect a person with a damaged immune system.

Pandemic
A disease that extends over an exceptionally large area, for

example, across continents, and affects large parts of the population.

Parasite
An organism that lives in or on another living organism at the expense of the latter.

Parotid gland
A salivary gland in front of the ear.

Pelvic, pelvis
The pelvis is a basin-shaped cavity surrounded by bone at the lower end of the torso or body trunk.

Platelet
The smallest type of blood cell, which is necessary for blood clotting. A platelet deficiency can cause bleeding disorders.

Pneumocystis carinii **pneumonia (PCP)**
A disease caused by the micro-organism *Pneumocystis carinii*. Symptoms include increasing breathlessness, dry cough and fever.

Prophylaxis
Therapy or intervention used to prevent a disease or infection.

Protease
An enzyme able to hydrolyse proteins and peptides by proteolysis and, thereby, allow viral particles, released from one human cell, to become mature and infect other cells in the body.

Protease inhibitors
A class of anti-HIV drugs that inhibit the protease enzyme and thus prevent viral particles from maturing.

Protozoa
Microscopic, unicellular animals.

Radiotherapy
Treatment with X-rays, usually in order to kill cancer cells.

Reflexology
A system of massage though reflex points on the feet, hands and head, used as an alternative therapy.

Retinitis
Inflammation of the retina (the back of the eye), which can cause visual blurring or the sudden appearance of blobs that appear to float in front of the eye (floaters).

Retroviruses
A family of viruses, including HIV, that contain their genetic material in a form called RNA.

Reverse transcriptase
An enzyme that converts viral RNA into DNA. Once DNA has formed, HIV can become integrated into the chromosome of a human cell and remain there for the life of that cell.

RNA
Ribonucleic acid, which is present in all cells of the body and acts as a messenger, carrying instructions from DNA to form proteins.

Salmonella
A bacterium that causes diarrhoea.

Semen
Reproductive fluid of men.

Seroconversion
The development of certain antibodies that can be detected in the circulation. In an HIV-infected patient, seroconversion relates to the production of anti-HIV antibodies.

Serum
The yellowish fluid that remains after the blood has been allowed to clot.

Shingles
A disease resulting from the acute reactivation of varicella zoster virus in those who have had chickenpox previously. The symptoms are a painful, blistery rash on the body.

Sputum
The material expelled from the respiratory passages by coughing or clearing the throat.

Suppressor (T8) cells
A group of cells that suppress or slow down growth of invading organisms such as bacteria, viruses or fungi.

Symptomatic
Patient presenting with physical or subjective changes that may indicate a specific disease.

Thrush
See candidiasis.

Toxoplasma, toxoplasmosis
A parasite that may be present in poorly cooked food or cat excreta. Disease caused by this parasite is called toxoplasmosis.

Transmission of HIV
The way in which you catch HIV infection.

Tuberculosis (TB)
A disease caused by the bacterium *Mycobacterium tuberculosis*, which causes cough, weight loss, fever, night sweats and fatigue.

Tumour
A swelling caused by an abnormal cell multiplying to produce millions of cells that form a lump. A tumour may or may not be malignant.

T-4 (CD4) lymphocytes
Cells of the immune system that co-ordinate the body's response against infection.

Vaccine
A substance designed to provide protection against infection from a specific disease.

Vaginal sex
Sexual intercourse involving penetration of the penis into the vagina.

Varicella zoster virus (VZV)
A virus of the herpes family, which causes chickenpox and shingles.

'Window period'
This is a period of up to 3 months between the time someone is exposed to HIV and the time that its presence in the body will show up on a test.

Index

JC virus, 22

Kaposi's sarcoma (KS), 23
    (*see also* Tumours)

Lamivudine, 30
Leukoplakia, 20
Lipodystrophy, 32
Lymphoma, 23
    (*see also* Tumours)

MAI, *see* Mycobacterial infections
Maintenance therapy, 35
MCA, *see* Mycobacterial infections
Measles in HIV-positive children, 48, 50
Measles, mumps and rubella (MMR) vaccine, 49
Meningitis, 21
Menstruation unaffected in women with HIV, 43
Miscarriage in women with HIV, 43
MMR, *see* Measles, mumps and rubella
Mortality, 7, 61, 63
Mortgage issues, 56–57
Mother-to-child route of transmission of HIV, 9, 43–44, 45, 47
Mycobacterial infections, 21–22, 35

Needlestick injury, 14
Nelfinavir, 30
Neuropathy, 32
Nevirapine, 30, 44
Non-nucleoside reverse transcriptase inhibitors (NNRTIs), 29–30, 32
'Non-nukes', *see* Non-nucleoside reverse transcriptase inhibitors
Norvir®, *see* Ritonavir
Nucleoside analogue reverse transcriptase inhibitors (NRTIs), 29–30
'Nukes', *see* Nucleoside analogue reverse transcriptase inhibitors
Numbers of cases of HIV infection, 1, 7–8, 41, 61

Opportunistic infections, 20, 21–23
Oral sex, 9, 65

PCP, *see* Pneumocystis carinii pneumonia
PCR, *see* Polymerase chain reaction

Crixivan® is a registered trademark of Merck Sharp & Dohme Limited.

Agenerase®, Epivir®, Retrovir® and Ziagen® are registered trademarks of Glaxo Wellcome.

Hivid®, Fortovase® and Invirase® and Viracept® are registered trademarks of Roche Products Ltd.

Norvir® is a registered trademark of Abbott Laboratories Limited.

Sustiva® is a registered trademark of DuPont Pharma.

Viramune® is a registered trademark of Boehringer-Ingelheim Limited.

Videx® and Zerit® are registered trademarks of Bristol-Myers Squibb Pharmaceuticals.